VALLEY CARE ASSOCIATION
of SEWICKLEY, PENNSYLVANIA

VALLEY CARE ASSOCIATION
of SEWICKLEY, PENNSYLVANIA

Aging with Comfort and Dignity

ALISON CONTE & JANICE JELETIC

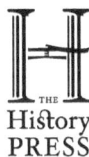

THE
History
PRESS

Published by The History Press
Charleston, SC
www.historypress.com

Copyright © 2020 by Alison Conte and Janice Jeletic
All rights reserved

Front cover, top right image: Nursing home resident Dr. Regis J. Ging enjoyed a visit from his son and daughter-in-law, David and Donna Ging. *Courtesy of Valley Care Association.*

First published 2020

Manufactured in the United States

ISBN 9781467143424

Library of Congress Control Number: 2019951265

Dedicated to Alice Hays and Reverend Russell W. Turner, who started it all, and to the seniors of the Sewickley Valley, especially those in our care.

We were community members who cared about the welfare of others.
It was just people helping people, with Valley Care as the connecting thread.

—Valley Care Association Newsletter, 2010

CONTENTS

Contents

FOREWORD

Volunteerism, philanthropy and nonprofit organizations have been unique and essential pillars of American communities since the founding of our country. These pillars have identified community and human service needs, formed structures designed to address these needs and financed these structures, leading to improvement in the overall health and well-being of the communities served.

The historical impact of the melding together of the three pillars to address social, cultural, health, educational and poverty challenges is massive—and an indispensable factor in the formation of the values that define the ideal community. The history of the Valley Care Association (VCA) vividly illustrates how a sincere, caring and committed community can—through the combination of volunteerism, philanthropy and a nonprofit organization—successfully address a community's needs.

Some have argued that classical volunteerism is threatened in our current highly mobile, digitally directed, social media–dominated culture; that philanthropy has become corporatized; and that true nonprofit entities are not economically sustainable. While it is true that our culture is not that of 1980, it is also true that the millennial (born in 1981–96) and generation Z (born in 1995–2010) generations will define a new form of community involvement that will be based on the culture that defines their day-to-day lives.

The societal challenges will be equally important, and communities of volunteers will organize to address these challenges. The fundamental principles that are illustrated in this monograph and characterize the forty-year success of the VCA will serve to guide those who identify a community need, develop a vision designed to address the need and build a strategy to implement a plan and finance the entity.

The history of VCA defines and illustrates a set of universal principles that VCA and many other human services entities have applied in a disciplined and objective manner to achieve long-term success. They are:

1. Define precisely the community need
2. Energize and engage the entire community of interest
3. Confirm the community need quantitatively
4. Establish a structure able to create a vision, goals, strategic plan and budget
5. Build a solid and sustaining financial base
6. Hire committed professionals to build and operate the entity
7. Preserve the mission by accepting the changing reality of the community and build new tactics to achieve the goal
8. Modify the strategy and identify new operational partners as challenges change
9. Preserve endowment capital and honor the philanthropy that allows dreams to become reality
10. Identify and mentor new leaders and stay engaged in the larger human services community

The application of these principles does not guarantee the success of a human services initiative but will serve to guide a group of volunteers that identifies a community need and seeks to address the need in an organized manner.

The real essence of VCA is its volunteers and philanthropists, who through steady and devoted loyalty, have ensured that VCA will continue to meet the mission of its founders. This publication celebrates the vision, commitment, energy and unselfish service that hundreds of persons have offered over the past forty years. The true tale of this very special organization is to be found in the appreciative stories that affected families have recounted, the comfort that dedicated staff have provided and the added touch that volunteers have offered to patients and families. These have energized VCA's history.

All across the United States, caring communities are banding together to accept the responsibility for the well-being of their members. It is our hope that VCA's story will encourage and support the many volunteer-based nonprofits that are striving to make communities special for all citizens.

As we strive to define a role for VCA for the next generation, our leadership remains committed to the principles that have brought us to this point. This same discipline and focus will enable VCA to continue to fulfill its mission of serving our seniors and their families.

Daniel Brooks, MD
James Lamperski, CFP
William Ringle
VCE Board History Committee

PREFACE

F irst and foremost, Valley Care is the story of community. A community that had a vision to take care of its own. A community that came together, found strong leadership, remained focused and accomplished its goal.

When we were first awarded this assignment, Alison had the greater knowledge of the organization as a resident of the area and as a former employee of both Sewickley Valley Hospital and the *Sewickley Herald*. Over the years, she had met and worked with many of these people, reporting on events connected with Valley Care.

Growing up in nearby Avalon, Janice was aware of the Masonic Village and knew that it offered various living options for seniors. She had visited the facility to see members of her church who were unable to attend worship services, and she was acquainted with the services and mission of Lutheran SeniorLife.

Because both of us had experienced the emotions and frustrations of caring for aging parents, we were intrigued by the idea of chronicling the history of a community-based program that cares for the elderly. As we met with current board members and heard their passion, we were hooked.

So began our journey of meetings, interviews and site visits. As we delved into the history of the Valley Care Association and met many of the people who contributed to it, we developed a kinship with their vision, struggles and achievements.

As the months passed, and two dozen boxes of documents were explored and summarized, we probably became the two people who were most knowledgeable about how Valley Care came to be, how it thrives and how it has changed to become what it is today. This is the understanding that we want to share with you through this book.

What we learned was that the people who founded and continue to support Valley Care are no ordinary group. What stands out is how thorough and meticulous they have been in every detail. They were—and continue to be—good stewards and caring individuals who truly want the best possible solutions for seniors in the Sewickley Valley area.

Valley Care Association has been a professionally run, impressive organization from the beginning—one that has brought credibility to its programs and quality care to the seniors it seeks to serve. It's been a privilege to research and write this story.

We want to thank the current board for entrusting us with this task. We thank the people along the way who shared their memories, experiences, perspectives, documents and pictures. And we encourage anyone who reads this book to participate in some manner.

After all, we all aspire to one day enjoy our golden years with the dignity and independence that Valley Care Association has sought for the seniors in its care.

—Alison Conte and Janice Jeletic

1

In the Beginning
There Was Sewickley

If there hadn't been a Valley Care Association, there wouldn't have been a nursing home, and there wouldn't have been Masonic Village retirement community with all the services and housing options they offer today.
—Mary Hays Mathews, director of social services and admissions for Valley Care Nursing Home

Sewickley, Pennsylvania, is a town on the Ohio River that calls itself a village.

Those who live in and around Sewickley cherish their history and value their community with a genteel ferocity. Among the townships and boroughs that nestle along the northeast bank of the Ohio River and extend up into the hills, this is a community that is unique for many reasons.

Sewickley developed in an ideal spot along several major transportation corridors. Many of the first settlers in the late 1790s were farmers, but some of them operated inns to accommodate steamboat travelers.

Respectability and a sense of community first came to the Sewickley Valley in 1837–38, when two private schools were founded: Edgeworth Female Seminary and Sewickley Academy (then for boys only and still operating today as a coeducational institution). The railroads arrived in 1851, transforming this rural community into a desirable place to live within commuting distance to Pittsburgh.

Citizens met to consider a name for their town in 1840, choosing Sewickleyville. It was incorporated as Sewickley on July 6, 1853. The

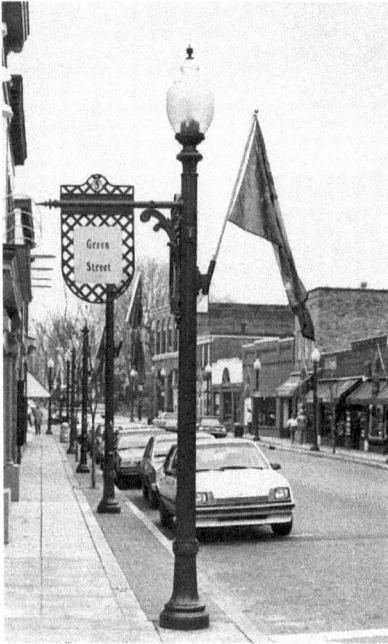

The village of Sewickley has a small-town feel that encouraged community spirit. *Courtesy of Sewickley Valley Historical Society.*

popular story is that the local Assiwikales Indian word *Sweekly* meant "sweet water" and referred to maple tree sap.[1]

The construction of the Sewickley Bridge in 1911 united the Valley with Coraopolis on the other side of the Ohio River. Soon the tracks of the railroad made way for highways—specifically, Ohio River Boulevard, a major artery also known as State Route 65, which stretches between Pittsburgh and the northwestern counties of the region. Inns and hotels accommodated travelers heading west to Ohio and beyond.

The industrialists—steel and coal barons—built grand country homes in Sewickley, Sewickley Heights and Edgeworth during the 1900s. They took the train out from smoky Pittsburgh to weekend and summer retreats on these idyllic, tree-lined riverbanks.[2]

Their household staffs, from cooks to chauffeurs, lived in the center of the town—still known as the Village—with the "merchant class." Some had houses in Leetsdale, Glenfield, Hays and Osborne, or "across the river" in Moon Township and Coraopolis. In time, professionals, retailers, business owners, IT entrepreneurs and professional hockey and football players discovered the area, diversifying the population.

The walkability of Sewickley Village was appealing to those who liked to run into their neighbors during an evening stroll. Even into the 1970s, many of Sewickley Valley's women didn't work outside the home, instead partaking in "society." They joined garden clubs, the Child Health Association, the Union Aid Society, the Sewickley Valley Hospital Auxiliary and other charitable organizations. These were people who were willing to give their time and treasure to support those who were less fortunate. They felt a responsibility to meet societal needs, particularly when government programs did not do so.

In 1978, the community found a new cause to join, champion, celebrate and support financially: Valley Care Association (VCA). VCA held out a loving hand to the area's oldest residents, giving them care close to home with respect and compassion.

Over the last forty years, VCA has operated a nursing home and two adult day care centers, improved access and safety for the elderly at home and given financial support to the efforts of other community programs for older adults.

ONE FAMILY'S LEGACY

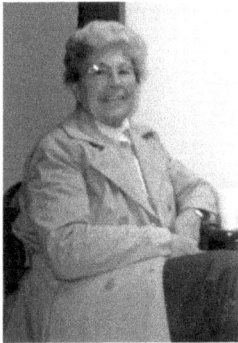

Alice Hays. *Courtesy of Valley Care Association.*

One Sewickley resident, Alice Hays, was instrumental in getting the idea of a community nursing home off the ground. In the mid-1970s, Hays was searching for a nursing home for her husband, John. He was in his late 50s and was suffering from early-onset Alzheimer's.

"There were no services for the elderly demented in the Sewickley Valley area at that time," Mary Hays Mathews, Alice and John's daughter, said. "There were no adult day care services, and Alzheimer's was still new and not talked about. My dad was eleven years older than my mother, and she had seven children to raise."

Hays needed help but didn't want her husband living far away. Finding so little care for the elderly nearby, she came to believe that this was a service that was missing in her hometown. She soon found that there were others who felt the same way.

LOCAL MINISTERS BRING COMMUNITY GROUPS TOGETHER

On May 4, 1978, representatives of several community organizations received a letter from the Reverend Russell W. Turner of Saint Stephen's Anglican Church, Sewickley.

Turner was convener of the Sewickley Ministerial Association, a group that included ministers from a number of Sewickley churches. The reverend's letter said that the "Ministerial Association had sponsored two meetings to consider the question of establishing a nursing home in our local area. The consensus of those present was that an action program should be initiated."

This nursing home, according to the letter, would serve all eleven local boroughs and towns that comprised the Quaker Valley School District. Turner invited all of the area churches, service clubs and organizations for the elderly to participate in establishing an independent organization for the purpose of raising funds to build and run a nursing home.

Each sponsoring organization would have two representatives on the board and would be expected to share in the starting costs of incorporation—twenty-five to fifty dollars for each group. There would also be members at large.

A meeting was set for May 23, 1979, at 8:00 p.m. in a conference room on the fourth floor of Sewickley Valley Hospital (SVH). This meeting included representatives from the Union Aid Society, Ministerial Association, SVH, Senior Citizens Club of Sewickley and Friendship House.

On June 7, 1978, the meeting minutes of Union Aid Society reported on the ministerial meeting: "About 60 people attended, and it was decided there was a need for an incorporating committee. Virginia 'Ginny' Schroeder was appointed as Union Aid's representative on this committee."[3]

The Union Aid minutes from September 13, 1978, stated that "Union Aid suggested the name of Valley Care for the nursing home and this name was accepted."

On September 19, 1978, Turner wrote to lawyer Martin L. Moor Jr., and said that VCA was incorporated, and a meeting of the first board of directors would be held to establish the bylaws on September 28 at 8:00 p.m. at the hospital. The letter stated, "I would strongly urge each [representative] to do some advance thinking in regard to the final constitution of the board of directors and how any organization becomes a part of Valley Care Association, etc. It is most important for us to be thorough and careful at this stage."

"I was living in California," Mary Hays Mathews said, "And when I called my mother, she was always talking about these early morning meetings at the hospital, as they worked to establish Valley Care." Giving back to the community through health care services was a family tradition, according to Mathews. "Think of others before yourself was the family mantra," she said.

Alice Hays became a vice president of the VCA board, serving for a total of nine years. Sadly, the opening of the Valley Care Nursing Home came too late for her husband, John, who was one of the first people in the country to be diagnosed with Alzheimer's. Alice eventually found care for him at the Veterans Hospital in Aspinwall, where he died in 1982.

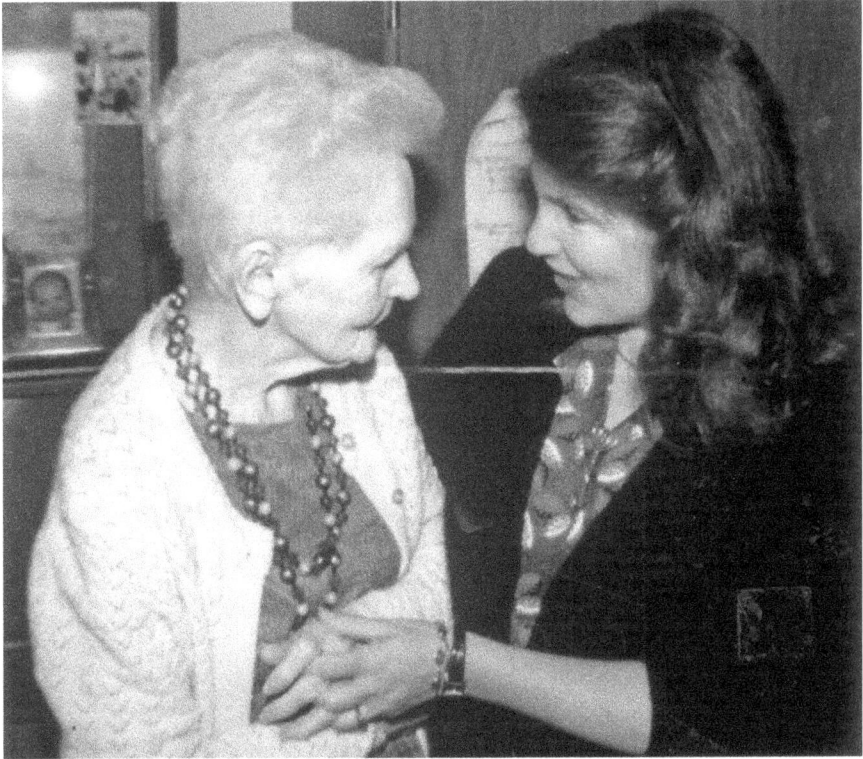

Anne Washburn, Valley Care Nursing Home resident, visits with Mary Mathews, director of admissions and social services for the nursing home. *Courtesy of Valley Care Association.*

A Need for Extended Care in the Region

"The groups that formed Valley Care were motivated by an absence of extended care services in the region," said Dan Brooks, MD, who served on the Valley Care Association and Valley Care Endowment boards.

"People who were aging and lived their lives in the Sewickley region wanted to create a comprehensive, continuous care alternative that afforded them the option to remain in the community through their lives," he said.

These facilities could also fill a need for nursing care generated by the shift to shorter hospital stays after illness or accident. Brooks, who was on the medical staff of SVH at the time, was very aware of how challenging it was for families to care for a profoundly dependent, senile or chronically ill parent or spouse at home.

"This was a time of limited government-based human services. There was a history—such as in the construction of the hospital—of addressing these issues locally and through private philanthropy," Brooks said.

FOUR GROUPS THAT AIDED SENIORS

Union Aid Society

Union Aid Society was a philanthropic organization formed in Sewickley in 1898. It was created by a group of women from local churches who came together to help neighbors. This union of church charities was a lifeline for area residents and provided financial aid and social services for many decades. Alice Hays volunteered as executive secretary.

Early on, Union Aid funneled charitable donations to those in desperate straits, giving milk and castor oil to babies; helping families through flu epidemics; and connecting people with nurses, cooks and housecleaners. In 1972, it built an eight-unit apartment building for low-income residents—housing that would expand to twenty-four apartments by 1988. Located on Centennial Avenue, these apartments were within walking distance of Sewickley Village, a boon for elderly residents.

As of 2019, Union Aid continued to offer housing and additional services for seniors and others in need, including:

- Referrals for home health-care personnel
- Registration assistance for eligible residents for transportation
- Financial aid for day care, summer camps, medical prescriptions, dental care and eyeglasses
- Help to pay for food, clothing, utility bills and rent

Friendship House

In 1951, Union Aid Society pioneered the Friendship House to provide housing to "genteel" elderly women. "It was for older ladies who had nowhere to go," said Eleanor Friedman, who served on the board of Union Aid in the 1980s. "They did not receive medical care but were expected to bathe and dress themselves and be downstairs for breakfast at an early hour."

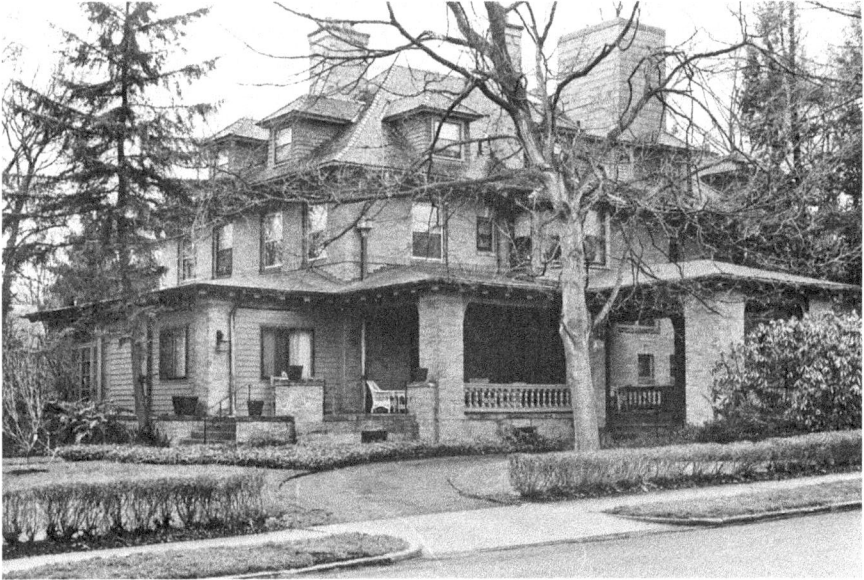

Friendship House. *Courtesy of Sewickley Valley Historical Society.*

Union Aid purchased a large house at 902 Centennial Avenue, formerly owned by Margaret Miller Book, for $22,500 in 1950. It was remodeled to create seventeen bedrooms, three new baths and a new kitchen, accommodating twenty people.

Friendship House was described as an "old folks' home" and was chartered as its own organization on June 14, 1951, licensed as a boardinghouse. The objective was to "own and operate a home for elderly people having no proper place to live and who deserve help."[4]

"It is to be a home for elderly residents of the Sewickley district. For many years the Union Aid Society has been conscious of the great need in Sewickley for such a home. The Union Aid is very pleased that it has been able to pioneer the start of such a home."[5]

Friendship House closed in February 1997, after forty-five years, having cared for 160 adults, including two men.

Sewickley Valley Hospital

Sewickley Valley Hospital was established in 1901, after citizens banded together to secure a charter and raise the funds to build it. The fourteen-bed hospital opened on July 20, 1907, on the east side of town against the hills of Sewickley Heights. It opened a school of nursing in 1916 and continued to flourish at the same spot for more than one hundred years. When funds were needed to improve technology or build additions, local residents gave generously.

George E. McCague, the first president of SVH, was Alice Hays's grandfather. His wife, Dorothy, established the first "family room"—what is now called a waiting room—at the hospital.

McCague explained his vocation and his family's legacy: "We are engaged in the work of intelligently alleviating human suffering and serving human life. There is no duty so imperative upon civilization."

Many hospital employees were also patients and lived in the area. They included Sewickley resident Mary Jane Williams, who worked in community relations for decades. "I've been so fortunate in the hundreds (maybe even thousands) of people I've met through SVH—my co-workers, the volunteers, clergy, auxiliary members, board members, doctors—many of whom have become good friends. I have a feeling of pride and gratitude, pride in my hospital and gratitude for being a part of it," Williams said.

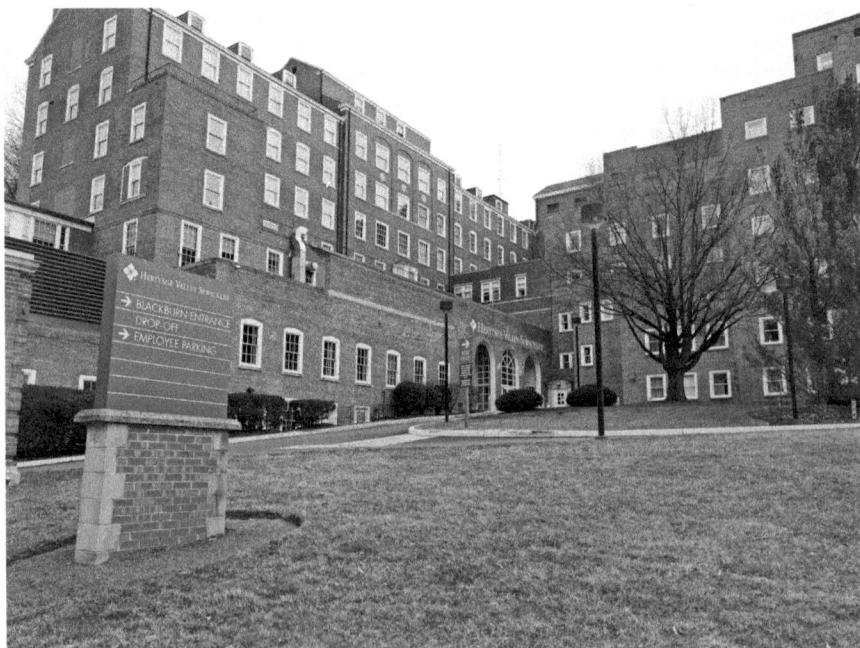

Sewickley Valley Hospital was a loyal supporter of VCA. *Courtesy of Valley Care Association.*

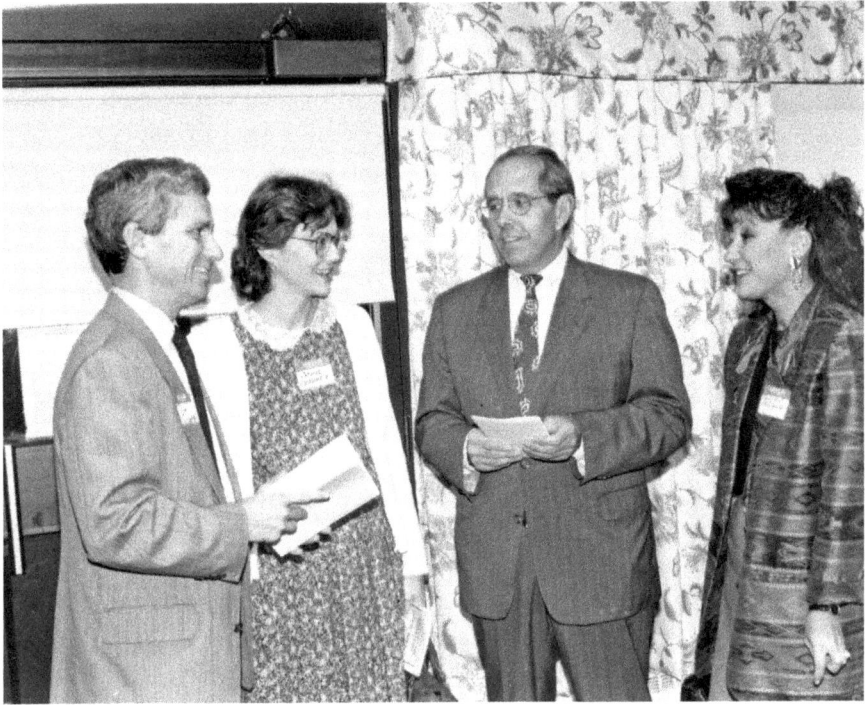

SVH Vice President and VCA board member Jim Cooper talks with Anne Ondrey, Dr. Robert Doebler and Danielle Zatezalo at a VCA members meeting. *Courtesy of Valley Care Association.*

In the early 1970s, SVH started a task force to determine how it could better serve the needs of the elderly in its service area of 87,000 people. The hospital was discharging an average of 101 patients each year directly to nursing homes, validating the need for a nursing home closer to Sewickley.

Hospital administrators considered converting the former SVH School of Nursing building into a nursing home, but projections showed that it could not be financially independent. Instead, the hospital started a home care nursing service and a Meals on Wheels food delivery program to serve older adults, as well as those who were ill or house-bound.

Led by SVH assistant administrator Marvin Wedeen, who became an active member of the VCA board, the hospital proved to be a valuable partner in establishing and supporting VCA. SVH medical staff tended to the health of VCA residents. Hospital leadership and employees contributed their knowledge and experience in health care and social services, forging an ongoing partnership with the nursing home and other VCA endeavors.

Senior Citizens Club of Sewickley

The Senior Citizens Club was a social organization for older adults that was first mentioned in the archives of the *Sewickley Herald* in 1968. The group initially met twice a month on Friday afternoons at Saint Paul's Lutheran Church in Sewickley. All senior citizens were invited to attend for fellowship, entertainment and refreshments.

The club often presented lectures from area residents. Topics ranged from new transcribing devices for the blind to a local couple showing slides of their vacation trip to Yellowstone Park. The group held a Christmas party each year, as well as an annual picnic and corn roast in the summer. Field trips included tours of Old Economy and other destinations.

The last notice of a club meeting in the *Sewickley Herald* was in 1991.

SETTING GOALS FOR A NEW ORGANIZATION

VCA's first membership meeting was held November 2, 1978, in a conference room of the hospital.

"The original board was twenty-five people," said David Nimick, who served as the first treasurer and continued on the board for seven years. The board included "five people from each of the [founding] organizations. It was a large board that eventually got whittled down."

"I became involved with Valley Care in the summer of 1978 when my wife, June, who is an active volunteer and trustee for Friendship House, asked me if I would help," Nimick said in a *Sewickley Herald* interview in 1981.

"It was always a geographically diverse board, with people from Sewickley Heights as well as Ambridge. We involved communities outside the boundaries of Sewickley borough," recalled Marvin Wedeen, who spent thirty years as a VCA board member.

Eleanor "Lannie" Gartner was involved with VCA for many years and served on the board from 1983 until 1985. Gartner said, "I lived in Moon Township in 1979. For Valley Care, I was the voice from 'across the river.'"

Gartner had worked as an occupational therapist at a hospital in Buffalo, New York. "I knew that there were too many people staying too long in the hospital to recover, at higher costs than were necessary. I could see that there was a need for a nursing home," she said.

"We were convinced that it was the responsibility of the community to have senior care services locally, so families could visit and the older adults could keep their own doctors," Nimick recalled.

"In Sewickley, we had some personal care homes that had nursing services for senior citizens. But we felt that this approach was limited in terms of quality and quantity. That led us to think about a nursing home. We decided we could raise money and borrow money to build one," Wedeen said.

The first membership meeting was conducted by Turner. Those present reviewed the bylaws, formed a nominating committee to choose a slate of officers and prepared publicity about VCA for the local newspapers. One of the first orders of business was to find a consultant who could coach them on the necessary steps to establish a nursing home.

The first article that mentioned VCA appeared in the *Sewickley Herald* on November 8, 1978:

> *Valley Care Association, a new nonprofit corporation, established to operate and maintain a nursing home in the Sewickley Valley area, began business November 2, 1978.*
>
> *Care for the aged will be a primary goal in planning. Ahead are decisions on location, size and design of a facility, feasibility studies, and the review of federal and state regulations concerning nursing home operation.*
>
> *At the November 2 meeting Dr. Sidney Selkovits, Thomas Neeley, and Paul Ramsey were chosen as a nominating committee. Mrs. William Colbert, David Nimick, Calvin Heinlen, and Mrs. Frank C. Schroeder, Jr., will serve on the Resolutions Committee.*
>
> *The group will meet next on November 16, at the SVH. Time of the meeting is 4:30 p.m.*

The twenty-five founding members of the VCA Board of Trustees were Frank E. Beall, Ralph Benz Jr., Mrs. William H. Colbert, Robert D. Duggan, Mrs. John A. Hays, Calvin X. Heinlen, Paul Hickox, Dr. Edward E. James, Mrs. B.F. Jones III, Mrs. Donald J. King, W. Neely Jr., David A. Nimick, Nathan W. Pearson, Mrs. Charles J. Ramsburg Jr., Paul D. Ramsey, Dr. Agnes S. Ronaldson, Mrs. Frank C. Schroeder Jr., Dr. Sidney Selkovits, G. Whitney Snyder, H. Alan Speak, James H. States, Reverend Jezreel Toliver, Reverend Russell W. Turner, Mrs. Allan W. Walter and Marvin M. Wedeen.

These individuals were an illustrious group, a who's who of Sewickley society. Board members throughout the years included active and retired leaders of industry and finance, local government officials, attorneys, real estate and investment professionals, doctors, academics, ministers, hospital administrators and nonprofit executives. Many of the members served on other local boards, guiding nonprofit organizations that supported

BRIDGE VOLUNTEERS FIND A NEW MISSION

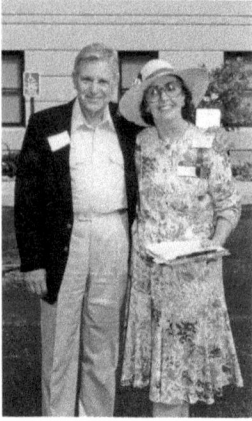

Marvin Wedeen and Gloria Berry were both volunteers for the Committee to Save the Sewickley Bridge in 1979. *Courtesy of Valley Care Association.*

Marvin W. Wedeen, assistant administrator for SVH, was a volunteer in 1977 with the Committee to Save the Sewickley Bridge. This group was formed after the Pennsylvania Department of Transportation closed the bridge, which spanned the Ohio River between Sewickley and Coraopolis, for safety reasons.

"We worked 60 hours a week on the bridge project. We went to Harrisburg to talk to the bureaucrats and the governor," said Sewickley resident Gloria Berry, another volunteer. By 1979, the committee had convinced the state that a replacement bridge was a necessity. "That project created a group of community advocates who continued to meet yearly on the anniversary of the opening of the bridge," Berry said.

The bridge project gave these volunteers a taste of what they could accomplish. Many of these same volunteers would later become involved with VCA.

churches, garden clubs, environmental concerns, literacy, fitness, health care, the arts and education.

On November 16, 1978, the group adopted bylaws and elected officers: Reverend Russell Turner, president; Allan Speak, first vice president; Alice Hays, second vice president; Elizabeth Walter, secretary; and David Nimick, treasurer.

The group met three more times in 1978. One meeting included a presentation by architects and several consultants who "addressed matters to consider when setting up a health care facility," according to the minutes. Small committees were formed with specific areas of focus: concept and policies, professional services, fundraising, public relations, sites and study of operating nursing homes.

On March 20, 1979, VCA received a certificate of exemption from income tax from the IRS. It was organized as a nonprofit corporation under the laws of the Commonwealth of Pennsylvania to receive tax-deductible contributions.

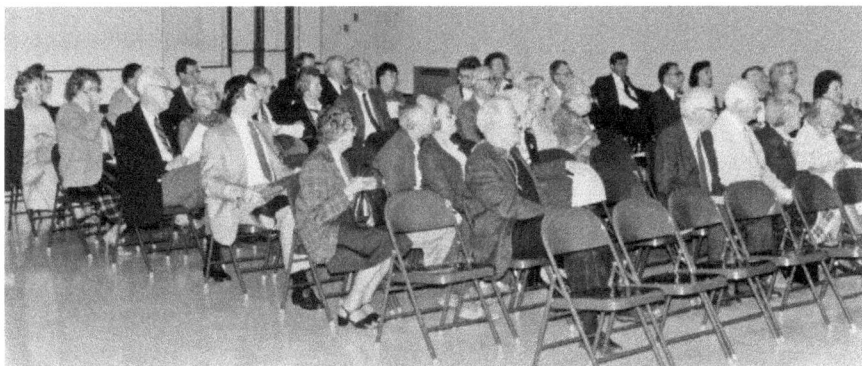

VCA members attend the first VCA annual meeting in 1979. *Courtesy of Valley Care Association.*

GAINING GROUND AND MEMBERS

Through publicity and mailings, members of churches and other area residents were invited to join VCA. Members made contributions of $15 or $25 each year, but membership neither conferred any special privileges nor secured a place on the waiting list to the nursing home. "You didn't have to be a member. That was just a way of getting people to support the idea [of building a nursing home]," said Wedeen. "Mostly they contributed $5 to $25. One family sent $5,000. Fortunately, we had some very wonderful people in Sewickley and Sewickley Heights with money who were able to help us set up in the beginning."

DEFINING THE MISSION AND GOALS

VCA's board needed to determine the community-based solutions that it would offer to older adults to enable them to remain active and engaged as they aged while remaining close to family and friends. They looked at the entire continuum of care that older adults needed, focusing on:

- A nursing home for long-term care and short-term rehabilitation
- An assisted-living facility
- An independent-living or retirement community
- Adult day services to provide socialization and structure
- Referral services to connect families to care and housing resources

The board intended to serve the needs of all residents, including those who could not easily afford care and those who needed specific services to cope with mental disorientation. VCA hoped to build the best possible facility without the use of government funding, relying instead on its neighbors' strong sense of community and generosity.

The proposed nursing home would draw customers from SVH's service area of approximately 122,000 people. This service area was composed of twenty towns in the Quaker Valley School District area, the airport area and southern Beaver County: Aleppo, Aliquippa, Ambridge, Baden, Bell Acres, Coraopolis, Crescent, Economy, Edgeworth, Glenfield, Harmony, Haysville, Hopewell, Leet, Leetsdale, Moon, Osborne, Sewickley, Sewickley Heights and Sewickley Hills.

Patterns of Aging in America

Against this backdrop of local community concern and activism, the United States was facing a huge challenge with an aging population that required enormous resources and creative solutions.

In 1900, the United States had 3.1 million people age sixty-five and older, composing about 3 percent of the nation's population. In those years, life expectancy at birth was forty-seven years. It rose to sixty-eight years by 1950 and to seventy-seven for men and eighty-two for women by 1975. Age sixty-five was chosen as the threshold to receive Social Security because, it was thought, only a few years of this support would be required.

When VCA was refining its mission in 1980, those over age sixty-five accounted for about 7 percent of the population, or 24 million people. According to a demographic study by Neil L. Gaynes and Associates of Chicago regarding this population:

- One in three was responsible for the care of an aged parent
- About 30 percent were over age seventy-five
- 90 percent had a chronic illness
- 40 percent had limitations imposed on their daily activities
- 5 percent were considered "home bound"
- 7 percent required a mechanical aid for mobility
- Nearly 70 percent owned their own homes
- One-fourth had incomes at or below federally defined poverty levels

- Another 25 percent had incomes more than $10,000
- Nearly all were covered by Social Security and used Medicare to partially cover the costs of health care

Aging Americans with the means to downsize their homes and responsibilities could move to a retirement community or independent-living facility. There, the average age was seventy-nine, with 25 percent of residents younger than seventy-five and 25 percent older than eighty-five. The eighty-five and older age group was the fastest growing segment of the U.S. population.

An alternative to a retirement community was a nursing home, or other home for the aged, where the average age was just over eighty-one years old, with 14 percent of those residents younger than seventy-five. The population in nursing homes was 85 percent female because more women lived to the age when they needed care.

In 1980, U.S. public and private spending for nursing home care was $22 billion, which rose to $53.1 billion in 1990[6] and to $162.7 billion by 2016 (including retirement community care).[7] In 1977, the average annual adjusted and unadjusted price of private nursing home care in the United States was $8,645.[8] In 2016, the typical annual cost of nursing home care was $82,000, which was nearly three times the annual income of most seniors.[9]

The majority of the spending went to care for long-term patients, with nursing homes also providing care for those recovering from physical illnesses, broken bones and reversible mental illness.

Family proximity remained important. Nearly 90 percent of the elderly were within a one-hour drive from their children, with two-thirds within walking distance.

During the 1980s, services were expanding to provide the elderly population with programs to help them live independently in the community. These included occasional or regular social activities, home-delivered meals or nursing care, housekeeping assistance and transportation to doctors' appointments and errands, as well as comprehensive adult day care with health care, meals and therapy.

In Pennsylvania, 1.3 million elderly made up 11 percent of the population in 1980, slightly higher than the national average.

Within the SVH service area, 9.2 percent, or 13,500 people, were older than sixty-five, and 4,000 of these were seventy-five or older. Families in Edgeworth, Sewickley Heights and Sewickley Hills had average family incomes of more than $15,000. Nine other communities had average family incomes of $7,000 or less.

BOARD MEMBER PROFILE: MARVIN WEDEEN

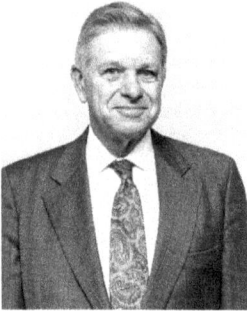

Marvin Wedeen. *Courtesy of Valley Care Association.*

Born January 3, 1926, Marvin Wedeen began his career in the food industry, ended it in health care and spent more than thirty years on the board of VCA. He was one of the first people to move into the retirement community of Masonic Village, fulfilling his own legacy.

In November 1971, Wedeen became assistant administrator at SVH. He lived at the Sewickley YMCA across the street from the hospital and ate all his meals at the hospital cafeteria until his family moved from White Plains, New York, in January 1972.

In 1980, the *Sewickley Herald* selected Marvin Wedeen as the 1979 Man of the Year for his work to save the Sewickley Bridge, writing, "Every good cause needs a catalytic agent and, fortunately, when Sewickley learned it was in danger of losing its bridge, Marvin Wedeen was on the scene. He has been described by a fellow member of the Committee to Save the Sewickley Bridge as the prime mover of the bridge crusade....His position as assistant administrator of SVH has been his springboard in serving to motivate the formation of other groups to improve life at the local level, including the hospital and ambulance authorities and the Valley Care Association. In all his community work he has advocated setting the goal and striving realistically toward attaining it. He is a quiet-spoken achiever who bears out the adage that action speaks louder than words."*

"Marvin was well organized, always prepared and persistent," said Dan Brooks. "He was a keenly observant advocate for the causes that he espoused in the interest of the community."

---

* *Sewickley Herald*, February 27, 1980.

This data translated into a measurable need for 680 long-term nursing home beds for the seventy-five and older population. When the people in these communities came together to create VCA, an organization that would furnish this care and fill this previously unmet need, they transformed the way services for the elderly were delivered in the Sewickley area.

2

Early Research Defines
the Need and Opportunity, 1978–80

To plan and build a nursing home which will offer three levels of care—skilled nursing, intermediate and custodial—and to accept patients who are receiving Medical Assistance payments.
—VCA mission, 1979

Valley Care Association trustees felt strongly that a marketing study should be undertaken before any other commitments were made to "prove that you need a nursing home before you make any commitments." They asked the membership for additional contributions to pay for a feasibility study.

In February 1979, VCA hired Patricia Loubeau, a graduate student at the University of Pittsburgh Health Services Administration, to make a demographic study of the area served by Sewickley Valley Hospital (SVH). Loubeau's survey found an unmet need for 173 skilled beds and 96 intermediate care beds and a need for nonresident services, such as finding care, community education, coordination of service delivery, enabling care, transportation, information and referral.

In March 1979, VCA distributed a questionnaire to area churches and received responses from 314 families. Fifty-three people said that a family member had an immediate need for a nursing home, and sixty-five people said they would need it in the future. Of these, forty-five lived in the Sewickley area.

An In-Depth Market Analysis

The board commissioned a demographic marketing study in June 1979, on the needs of the elderly and the availability of services for them. The board hired Neil L. Gaynes and Associates of Chicago at a cost of $26,700. At the time, VCA had a balance of $3,485.78 in its accounts and pledges or donations of $24,750. Agreeing to spend this amount showed the board's strong faith in its ability to continue to raise funds. It was also a demonstration of how important the organization felt it was to rely on the expertise of professional consultants to guide it through this venture.

On December 13, 1979, Gaynes gave a brief summary of his report to the board. He said that services provided for the elderly in the area included health care, social activity, hotel services and management. He also reported that the average age of patients in nursing homes nationwide was eighty to eighty-two, that 75 percent of residents' costs were paid for by Medicare, Medicaid or some other third party, and that just 25 percent of residents paid privately.

Gaynes stated, "It should be recognized that the public image of frail and delicate elderly is, for the most part, a misconception. Less than five percent of the elderly population is, at any given time, found in a nursing home. Another five percent are considered home bound, and seven percent require some sort of mechanical aid for mobility."

Existing Facilities for the Elderly

The Gaynes study found an uneven distribution of services for the elderly in 1979. There were forty-nine long-term care facilities in Beaver and Allegheny Counties with a capacity of 7,300 people. Of these, 88 percent of the facilities were in Allegheny County. Only two of these facilities were in the SVH service area: Golfview Manor in Aliquippa with fifty-eight beds and Naugle Manor in Baden with nineteen intermediate care beds and no Medicaid residents.

Gaynes projected the primary and secondary service areas would need 680 long-term care beds for the four thousand people in those areas who were then older than seventy-five—about 520 beds for skilled nursing and 160 beds for personal care. He concluded that Valley Care could justify establishing 500 long-term beds with 80 percent for skilled nursing, filling any gaps in services with one of the following options for a nursing home facility:

- Option 1: A nursing home with less than 120 beds available at $700 to $800 a month with no entry fee and private pay with certification under Medicare if money ran out, requiring a $5.5 million to $6 million investment, not including the cost of the land.
- Option 2: A nursing home with 120 to 150 beds, offering skilled nursing care for the elderly dependent on Medicaid alone or in addition to private pay, requiring $5.2 million to $6.3 million.
- Option 3: Replacement housing for older people to move into when they were no longer able to be completely independent.

As the board debated its next steps, it returned to the original philosophy: to return every resident to the highest level of independence and ideally discharge them back home. The alternative was to support the resident at the highest level of freedom and dignity as possible within the confines of a facility.

The mission was always focused on serving the elderly, and spending was directed toward that objective. "We supported various projects along the way, but there were concerns that we were getting away from truly caring for seniors, which is what we wanted to do," Marvin Wedeen said.

Two key concerns were appropriateness and finances. The services offered were to fit into the available long-term care offerings without duplicating existing facilities. If VCA tried to offer too many services, it could drain its financial resources.

In January 1980, the board approved a motion to implement option 2, as outlined by the Gaynes Report, for a nursing home with 90 to 120 beds. The cost would be $25,000 per bed, or $3,775,000 for a 150-bed facility. Though 80 percent could be borrowed, the rest would be raised through a fund drive.

BUILDING FINANCIAL SUPPORT

As VCA's membership grew, its financial base solidified. During the first year, 1978–79, membership grew from 26 to 101, as individuals, churches and organizations joined the association. By September, VCA had 195 members. By the 1981 fiscal year, VCA's membership had grown to more than 300. The treasury grew through these contributions, as well as through grants and private donations. The fundraising goal was $2.8 million.

"We had a community that was very supportive and a few special people who had seed money," said Wedeen. "We raised $2 million and borrowed $6 million."

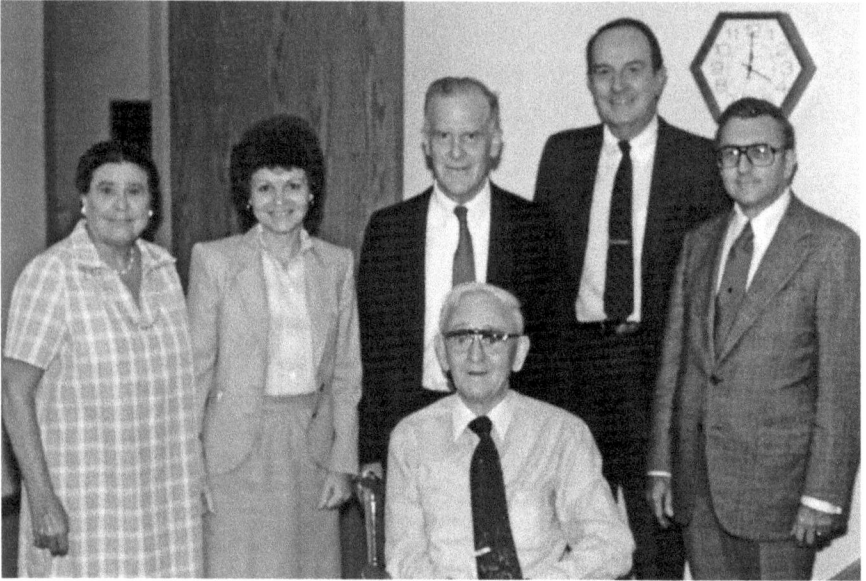

Elizabeth Walter, Judy Comer, David Nimick, Whitney Snyder and Gene March thank Dan Lessenberry (seated) for his contribution to the building fund. *Courtesy of Valley Care Association.*

In February 1981, David Nimick described the group's status in an article in the *Sewickley Herald*:

> *Now we have the necessary front-money to pay for the plans and financial feasibility studies to have the project reviewed by the Health Systems Agency,* [which] *must give approval to all hospitals and nursing homes before such facilities can be built anywhere in the United States.*
>
> *It's going to be a tight schedule, but we hope we can have our proposal ready for review by the Health Systems Agency by March 31. We've been having weekly meetings of the trustees and our professional consultants to try to meet the deadline because the agency only makes reviews at certain times of the year.*
>
> *Besides the $7,500 we raised from membership, 63 persons made substantial gifts, which went toward making up the $90,000 we needed for planning. The total cost of the project is estimated at $6 million with $1.5 million of that going for an endowment to provide for those who can't afford to pay the cost of the care themselves. The trustees don't want this to be a home just for those who can pay.* [10]

BOARD MEMBER PROFILE: G. WHITNEY SNYDER

G. Whitney Snyder was a founding member of VCA and was instrumental in making the nursing home a reality. He was a VCA trustee for eleven years, from 1978 until 1989 and was vice president from 1981 until 1988. He always gave generously to support the association and, by example, encouraged others to do likewise.

He chaired the committee to organize Valley Care Nursing Home's tenth anniversary celebration in 1994. As a collector and hands-on restorer of antique cars and carriages, he offered his 1910 Pierce and other antique cars to enliven many VCA community events.

A native of Sewickley Heights, Snyder served the borough as a councilman for forty years, thirty of those as president. Chairman of the board of Shenango Incorporated, Snyder also served on the boards of Sewickley Academy, Sewickley YMCA, Sewickley Heights Trust and Laughlin Children's Center.

Snyder's dream was to create a public park, nature center and historical center in Sewickley Heights. In the 1990s, Snyder and others donated five hundred acres of undeveloped land to Sewickley Heights Park, bringing its total size to one thousand acres. Several years later, Snyder donated another piece of land, formerly part of his family's Wilpen Farm, for the Fern Hollow Nature Center and the Borough of Sewickley Heights History Center.

In 2018, Sewickley Heights History Center was filled with items accumulated by Snyder. They included the Snyder family's 1899 Rockaway carriage and a 1929 Ford Model A.

Snyder died on January 16, 1999.*

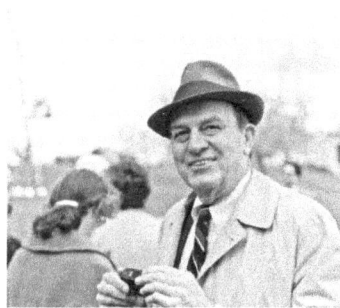

G. Whitney Snyder. *Courtesy of Valley Care Association.*

* *Pittsburgh Post-Gazette,* January 18, 1999, and January 25, 2001.

SUPPORT FOR MENTAL HEALTH SERVICES

The Staunton Farm Foundation was started in 1933 upon the death of Sewickley resident Matilda Staunton Craig McCready. In her will, McCready organized a foundation "to care for persons suffering from curable neurotic, mild mental, and kindred ailments." From 1933 until 1987, the Staunton Farm Foundation gave 290 grants of about $15 million to sixty organizations in the Pittsburgh area that provided such services.[11]

Because VCA intended to provide twenty beds for elderly patients with psychiatric disabilities, the board approached Staunton Farm for support. VCA's proposal and the foundation's response provided insight into VCA's plans and philosophy, expectations of how successful nursing homes should operate and how VCA's goals and operation measured up against other comparable projects.

In a letter to Staunton Farm Foundation on April 14, 1981, J. Robert Ferguson Jr., president of the VCA board from 1981 until 1987, said that VCA had "reached a critical point where major philanthropic support must be sought to move ahead with plans for a 120-bed nursing home."

He requested a grant of $500,000 for construction "that could pave the way for other major gifts" and "allow us to approach other foundations with confidence." Ferguson outlined the expected project costs as:

Land purchase	$450,000
Sewage development	$150,000
Construction	$3,000,000
Equipment	$220,000
Professional fees	$320,000
Construction management	$360,000
Contingencies	$400,000
Total	**$4,900,000**

Staunton Farm's reply encouraged the VCA board to submit a more formal, detailed grant request. In June, the board sent a fifteen-page proposal detailing the organization's philosophy and master plan (which included long-term goals to develop an assisted-living facility and a retirement community), financial statements, maps and drawings.

The proposal stated that the grant, and any future grants, would assure support for the psychological needs of three classes of VCA nursing home residents:

1. General residents who experienced anger, frustration and depression associated with moving from independent living into a nursing home
2. Confused and disoriented individuals and those with mental disabilities
3. Patients who experienced major trauma or surgery and required sub-acute psychological care

It was noted that while VCA did not intend to create a psychiatric hospital, "its close association with the Staunton Clinic (mental health services) of SVH would permit it to address the needs of residents afflicted with mental illness who may be considered 'unacceptable' in other nursing homes."

An Extraordinary Funding Opportunity

Staunton Farms requested that the proposal be reviewed by William P. Ferretti, a consultant to the foundation and a well-known national figure in matters of health policy and planning. Following his review, Ferretti urged approval of the grant saying, "Valley Care Association is presenting Staunton Farms with an extraordinary opportunity to fund a worthwhile project. The proposed Valley Care Association three-phase master plan holds great promise to place Valley Care Association and Staunton Farms in leadership positions nationally in the provision of nonprofit services to the elderly."

He described three factors that "ensure that the Valley Care Association is more advanced in its approach than traditional proprietary and government-owned nursing homes: it is a nonprofit organization, it has committed leadership, and it enjoys the strong support of the SVH."

He also recommended that Staunton Farms encourage VCA to develop alternative programs to ensure appropriate use of the nursing home. "It is widely held by many experts that the absence of support services in the community often forces some elderly people into nursing homes sooner than required…due to a general lack of formal alternatives to institutional care."

To avoid this situation, it was important that VCA move ahead immediately with its plans for a day care program for the elderly rather than delay it until the nursing home was built. "Day care programs can provide care for patients discharged from the hospital, respite care for families, social services, and medical services that could help the emotional disturbed elderly cope with the problems of daily living," Ferretti said.

He offered several recommendations to VCA:

- Have a volunteer program that will strengthen patient ties to the community
- Consider a management contract arrangement with SVH
- Employ a medical director with special interest in geriatrics and a geriatric nurse practitioner
- Keep pace with new knowledge in the field of elder care through a commitment to education and research in concert with local universities and colleges

VCA followed several of these recommendations, eventually starting a volunteer program and hiring a geriatric-oriented medical director. It opened an adult day care center in the Aleppo Township Municipal Building in May 1983, almost a year before the nursing home opened. (Read more about adult day services in chapter 7.)

THE OPERATIONS COMMITTEE CREATES A PLAN

VCA's operations committee was charged to evaluate management options, select a person or firm to accomplish the project and provide daily contact during the construction period. Chaired by H. Alan Speak, its first meeting was held on July 9, 1980.

At that meeting, the group agreed that the nursing home would have 75 percent shared rooms and 25 percent private rooms; skilled, intermediate and respite care; and a hospice facility for the terminally ill. It would also have twenty beds for the mentally confused or "disoriented."

The issue of whether or not to admit residents on Medicaid was resolved by the requirements of the Southwestern Pennsylvania Health System Agency, which would only approve new long-term beds in facilities with one-third Medicaid beds. The board recommended an endowment of $2 million, invested to earn interest, to pay for the cost of the beds that were not covered by Medicare.

In October 1980, the board approved the operation committee's recommendation. The minutes report a vote "to attempt the construction of a long-term care nursing home to serve the catchment area of the SVH as a first step in what it is hoped will later become a full retirement community offering independent living and assisted living, in addition to the skilled and intermediate services planned for the nursing home."

This three-phase master plan was envisioned to be accomplished over a four- to six-year period. In June 1981, the funding proposal to Staunton Farm included details about the timeframe for development:

- Initial: 120-bed nursing home with a wing to house up to twenty patients with psychiatric disabilities
- One year later: Transportation program for older persons in the community
- Two years later: Seventy-five to one hundred residential apartments with dining and recreational areas
- Four years later: New wing added to nursing home for increased outreach, such as adult day care, homemaker services and Meals on Wheels food delivery to homebound residents
- Two to four years later: New wing for sixty assisted-living units in conjunction with residential or outreach expansion
- Six years later: Twenty to fifty cluster residential units or additional assisted-living units

The goal was to have site, design, financial feasibility study and approval by the Health Systems Agency by the spring of 1981, with occupancy by 1983. The plan was delayed by about one year, with the nursing home eventually opening its doors in March 1984. The development of the full retirement community and assisted-living options proved to be a more difficult goal—one that would elude VCA for almost two decades.

Operations committee members visited nursing homes across southwestern Pennsylvania, including Baptist Homes in Castle Shannon, Mount Lebanon Manor and Redstone Presbyterian Home in Greensburg. They gained valuable insights from these visits, discussing with administrators a wide range of issues involving design, construction, entrance fees and the need for an advertising and public relations campaign to attract residents.

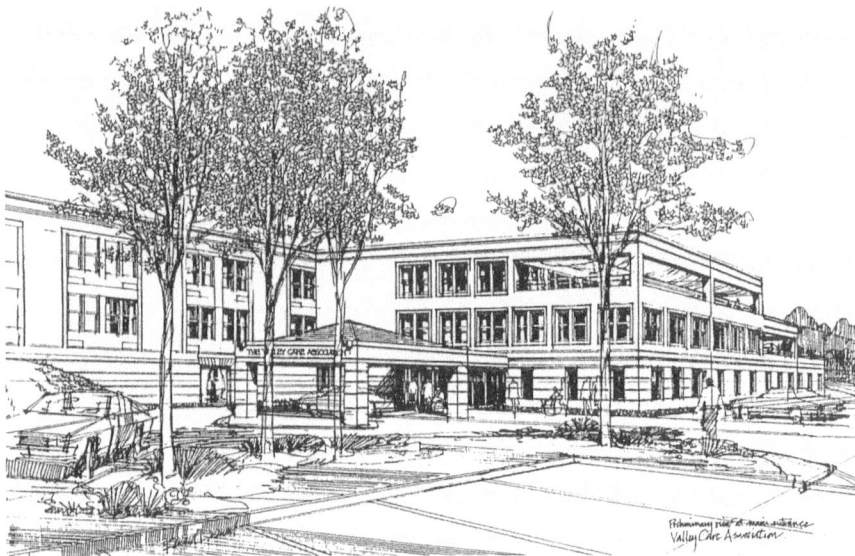

Architectural firm Reid-Ritchie made a preliminary sketch of the main entrance of the Nursing Home. *Courtesy of Valley Care Association.*

BUILDING A TEAM OF CONSULTANTS

One of the strengths of the VCA board was that they knew what they didn't know. As men and women with years of experience managing companies and serving other nonprofits, they knew the value of good consultants and didn't hesitate to call on them.

The operations committee advised the board to choose a local construction project manager who was affiliated with an architect and contractor, had expertise in nursing homes and had a strong commitment and willingness to work for the board. On December 10, 1980, the board approved hiring Reid-Ritchie and the Design Alliance, architects; Butcher and Singer, investment bankers; and Mellon Stuart Company, contractor/construction firm.

Other architectural and engineering firms mentioned in the groundbreaking program as contributing to the nursing home project were consulting engineers Betz-Converse-Murdoch Incorporated and Dodson Engineers, G.W.S.M. Incorporated, as well as R.M. Keddal and Associates, a land survey company.

Soon after, consultants were selected to provide financing and legal expertise: Mellon Mortgage Incorporated, to provide a Federal Housing Administration (FHA) insured mortgage; Arthur Young and Company, accounting; Property Development Associations, development attorney; and MacIntosh Associates, program consultants.

Crossgates Incorporated was selected as a managing agent to hire employees and manage the nursing home once it was operational. Crossgates was a developer that operated area nursing homes, including Murray Manor in Murrysville; Morgan Manor in Morgantown, West Virginia; Hillview in Coraopolis; and Mount Lebanon Manor in Mount Lebanon.

CONTINUING FINANCIAL SUPPORT

By September 17, 1981, $100,000 had been pledged by the board members. Instead of hiring an agency to run the fund-raising campaign, the development committee hired Elizabeth G. "Betts" Moore to be director of development. VCA opened an office in rent-free space at 434 Beaver Street, Sewickley, on November 20, 1981.

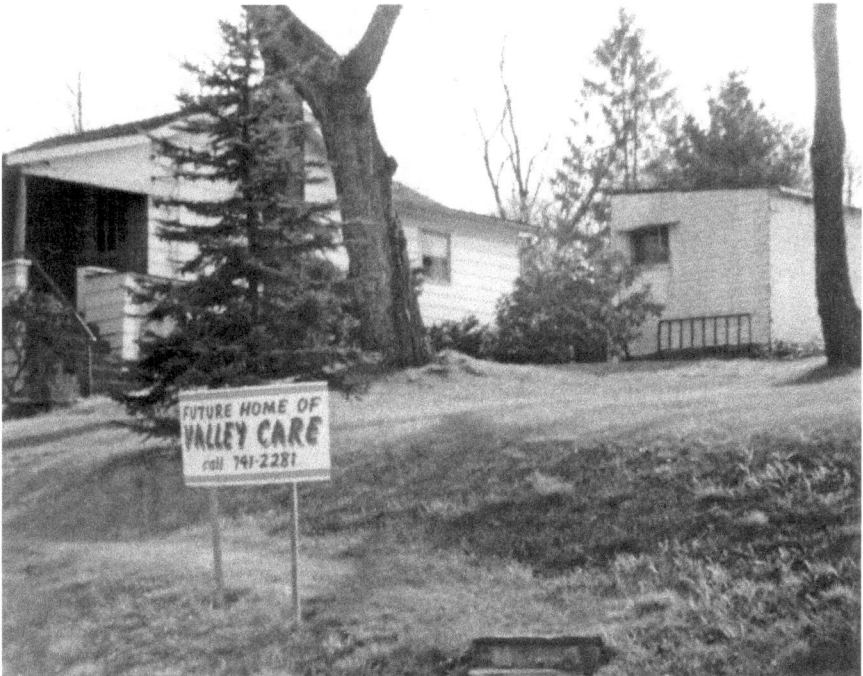

In 1983, this sign advertised the future home of Valley Care Nursing Home. *Courtesy of Valley Care Association.*

By this time, Mary Mathews had returned to Sewickley from Seattle with her son and daughter. While she was studying at Duquesne University and working part time at a Sewickley gift shop called Cheers, her mother (VCA board member Alice Hays) asked her to devote some time to "helping out Betts." So, Mathews became a part-time secretary in the fund-raising area.

Mathews and Moore initially worked out of borrowed office space in Sewickley and later from a little white house that was located on the Aleppo Township property, purchased by VCA for the nursing home.

GRANTS AWARDED, PLEDGES MADE

Staunton Farm Foundation approved VCA's grant application of $500,000, conditional upon VCA raising $2 million. The foundation's letter said, "In this way, we hope to ensure that most of the $2,800,000 you wish to secure from the private sector will be committed to the project."

As the grant was made in honor of Matilda Staunton McCready, the foundation said it would be "pleased to have you suggest a suitable memorial to her, perhaps the naming of a wing or some other suitable facility."

By December 1981, board president J. Robert Ferguson Jr. reported that VCA had received a $150,000 pledge from the W.P. Snyder Charitable Fund, as well as "modest and continuing support" from the Raymond John Wean Foundation and the Rust Foundation. Additional foundations were thanked in the 1983 ground-breaking ceremony program: Anne L. and George H. Clapp Charitable and Educational Trust, Cyclops Family Foundation, Howard Heinz Endowment, the Pittsburgh Foundation, Pittsburgh National Foundation and the Lucy K. Schoonmaker Foundation.

In 1982, as planning, design and construction commenced, fund-raising continued. Campaign totals, in cash and pledges, increased from $1,137,707 in February to $1,619,146 in October.

At the annual meeting in October 1983, the board announced that it had received contributions, pledges and interest of $2,059,702 toward its goal of $2.5 million. Of the $2.5 million, $1.9 million would be designated as equity and $600,000 as endowment funds. Of the equity funds, $344,000 was intended to be saved for the assisted-living and retirement projects. An FHA guaranteed bond issue was expected to yield $3,780,000.

EMPLOYEE PROFILE: BETTS MOORE

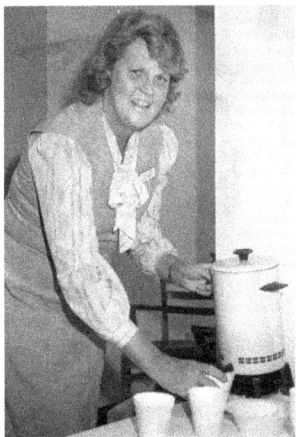

Elizabeth G. "Betts" Moore.
Courtesy of Valley Care Association.

Elizabeth G. "Betts" Moore was hired as director of development for VCA in 1981 and served until 1986.

Initially, she focused on the immediate need of fund-raising—a scope of work that broadened to all aspects of the organization—and she became executive director in 1984. She was involved with the nursing home and the adult day care center and was a "wonderful ambassador" for VCA in handling development, publicity and marketing.

In an article in the *Sewickley Herald* in 1984, Moore was quoted as saying, "I feel the pastoral setting of the Valley Care nursing home is conducive to the residents' recovery. We don't use the word patient here. We use the word resident. When someone is staying at Valley Care, we want him to feel this is his home."

"Betts has been the eyes, ears, and hands of Valley Care, focusing on whatever problems were of the greatest concern," said VCA president J. Robert Ferguson Jr., upon Moore's retirement on May 31, 1986. "It's hard to visualize Valley Care without her." He lauded her good-natured optimism, ability to work with others and faith in and concern for her fellow man.[*]

On May 21, 1986, Moore was honored at a dinner in gratitude for the "outstanding" manner in which she furthered the aims of VCA for six years. She retired due to health problems and died on November 28, 1986.

VCA named the Elizabeth G. Moore Scholarship Fund in her honor to give financial support for clients of the adult day care center.

---

[*] *Sewickley Herald,* June 4, 1986.

When the fund topped $2 million, Moore announced, "We've seen the successful completion of a goal at $2 million through the generosity of many individuals, foundations, and corporations, and we're pressing on toward $2.5 million."[12]

A solicitation letter to the community on November 30, 1983, asked recipients to pass along the names of "anyone who might be a potential client for either the nursing home or the adult day care center," as well as those who might be interested in living in the future retirement community.

Membership dues were received from 459 people that fiscal year, plus contributions from another 90. VCA neared its goal in late 1985, raising $2,450,000. More than 500 members, giving what they could to support the nursing home, contributed $4,000.

Just prior to the opening of the nursing home, Moore commented on the fund-raising campaign: "This was a community effort and we're proud. We got no government funding. Our $2.5 million was raised through community support and local foundations."[13]

After the nursing home and adult day care centers were opened, a strong endowment was needed to support the operations, which often ran at a deficit. Contributions were made to a fund to support those who could not fully afford to pay for care.

In a grant request proposal to Staunton Farm Foundation, VCA reaffirmed its commitment to "provide skilled and intermediate nursing home care to residents whose financial resources may not fully cover the cost of care. Valley Care would accept Medicare and Medicaid payments, recognizing that these would be less than the operating costs."

Members were solicited each year, with many renewing and others joining for the first time. Momentum grew and plans solidified. There were 236 members in 1979, 318 in 1980, 338 in 1981, 422 in 1982 and 583 in 1983. The number of renewing members fluctuated between 300 and 550 over the next ten years.

"It was the combination of a carefully drafted data-based plan with access to philanthropic resources and deep community support that defined the success of the campaign," said VCE board member Dan Brooks, MD.

3

Building a Nursing Home, 1980–87

Aging is a process, and not a disease or combination of entities
which can be cured, or against which one can be immunized.
—Neil Gaynes

When word got around that Valley Care Association was looking to purchase land, many properties were proposed and reviewed against the criteria set by the site selection committee, which was led by Paul Hickox.

The project required at least fifteen acres suitable for construction, including five for the nursing home and ten for the future retirement community. It would need appropriate sewage connections, utilities, zoning, easy access to major roads and highways—and to be close to Sewickley.

With this in mind, the committee considered several sites:

1. Twenty-four acres on Camp Meeting Road in Leet Township, near Sewickley Heights, across from D. T. Watson Rehabilitation Hospital, occupied by a par-three golf course
2. Sixty acres along Thorn Run Road in Coraopolis Heights, near Robin Hill Park, owned by Sewickley Valley Hospital and adjacent to its Moon Township medical offices
3. Fifteen acres of fairly level property at Backbone Road and Camp Meeting Road in Bell Acres Borough, owned by Sewickley Heights Estates (near Sewickley Heights Golf Club)

4. Quaker Valley School District property on Camp Meeting Road in Bell Acres
5. Staunton Farms site on Aliquippa Road, near Stoops Ferry Road in Moon Township, near Robert Morris College
6. Twenty-six acres on Merriman Road in Aleppo Township, across from the Route I-79 Industrial Park
7. Property on Ohio River Boulevard in Edgeworth and owned by Edgeworth, on Water Works Road with a view of the river

When all of the sites were reviewed by the Reid-Ritchie/Design Alliance architects, the first two were judged as having the most potential and were worth pursuing. The Leet Township site, described as the "Watson Home" property in the minutes, had eighteen buildable acres and a price tag of $450,000 (later developed as a housing plan on Chaucer Court, North and South). The Coraopolis Heights site was owned by SVH, and board members thought that it might be possible to get a long-term lease at no cost.

In December 1980, committee members discussed how the community would react to settling on the "other side of the river," demonstrating a long-held regional bias against crossing any bridge to do business. Board member Elizabeth Walter raised the philosophical question of where the customers would prefer to be. The preferences of potential benefactors were considered, but the hospital site's financial aspects were "hard to beat."

The board held three public meetings in April 1981, to inform the public about VCA's progress and plans. "In Coraopolis Heights, the survey results were not good, finding oil well drillings and high water," recalled board member Marvin Wedeen. "We considered the [Leet Township] land, but only had 30 to 60 days to make an offer, and that wasn't enough time to make a decision."

On April 27, 1981, VCA received a counteroffer on the Leet Township property, raising the price from $300,000 to $400,000. The April 30 committee minutes about that property reported that "land purchase, sewerage resolution, and zoning problems have yet to be overcome. Discussion ensued on the alternative Aleppo site potential being less initial cost [$250,000] and having fewer zoning and sewerage problems, but marketability of total program and philanthropy may be adversely affected."

On September 10, 1981, the committee voted to cease negotiations on the Leet Township site and proposed to secure the Aleppo Township site (number 6) for the project, despite reservations.

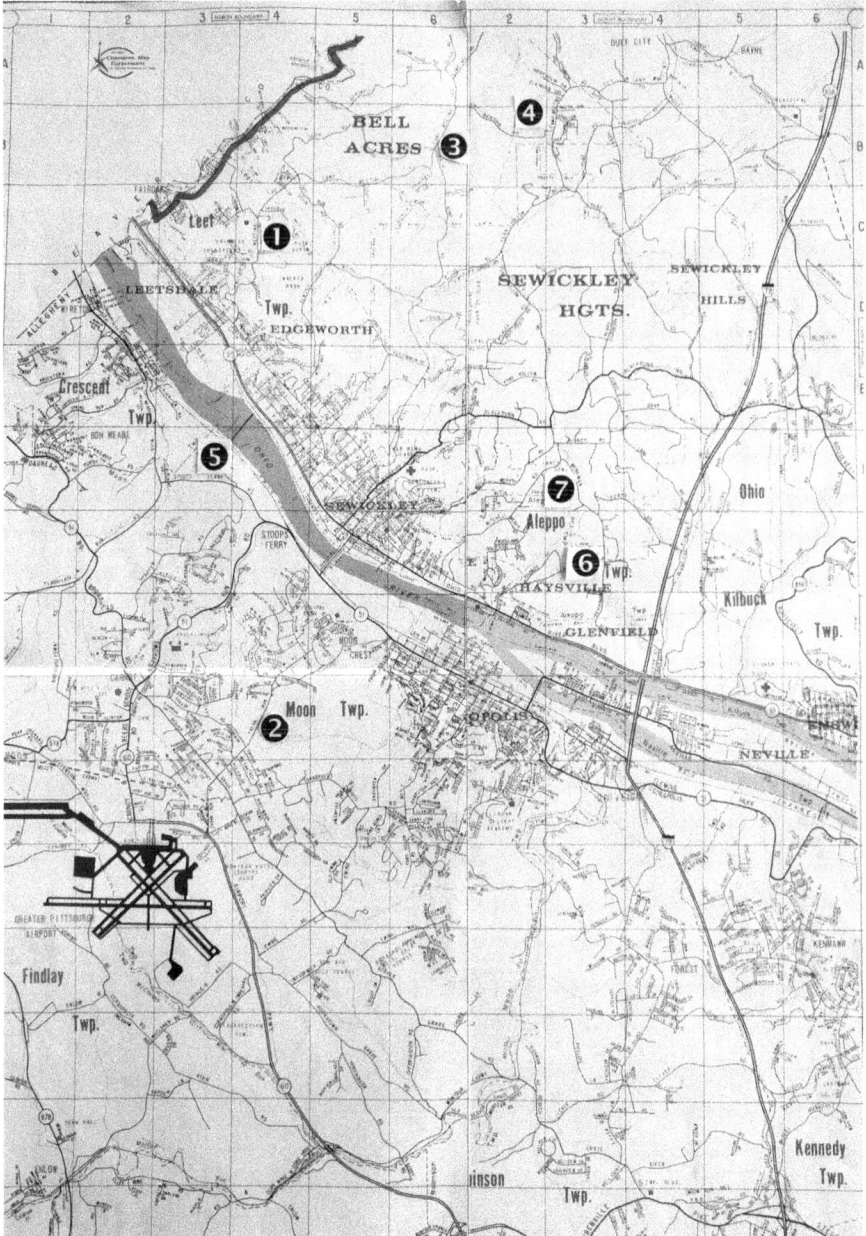

VCA considered seven sites for the Nursing Home. Numbers on the map correspond to the list in this chapter. *Courtesy of Pittsburgh Map Book, 1976.*

LOCATING IN ALEPPO TOWNSHIP

The Aleppo property was twenty-six acres on Merriman Road, a wooded site in Aleppo Township, two minutes from the intersection of I-79 and Ohio River Boulevard (State Route 65) and only seven minutes from SVH. "It was owned by a family in Coraopolis. We approached them and they agreed to sell us the land," said Wedeen.

The site was within twenty-five minutes of the farthest community in the service area. Seven acres would be used by the nursing home, with nineteen acres reserved for a sixty-bed assisted-living facility and two fifty-unit "congregate" living units, later referred to as retirement community housing.

Plans for the Aleppo site were shown at the VCA annual meeting on October 15, 1981. Construction would require compliance with Aleppo zoning ordinances covering subdivision and conditional uses of the property.

A public meeting was held on October 26 to request permission to build on Merriman Road. VCA president Robert Ferguson outlined the planned phases for development: nursing home, assisted-living facility and retirement apartments. "The major concern of the residents who attended the filled-to-capacity meeting…was one of taxes, since Valley Care is a nonprofit."[14]

Ferguson said that VCA would make payments to the municipality in lieu of taxes, as it "does not want to be a burden on Aleppo and was prepared to pay for the services it would be receiving, such as police and fire protection." Ferguson pointed out that Aleppo Township would earn funds from wage and occupation privilege taxes paid by employees. Finances and utility use also were discussed.

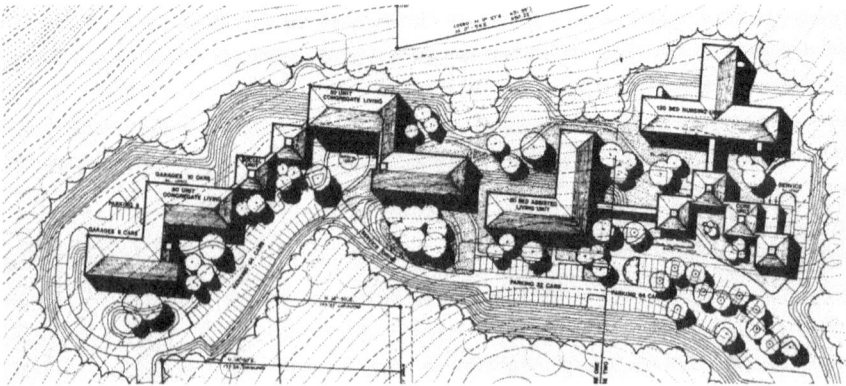

In 1981, VCA proposed this design to Aleppo Township, including the nursing home and future development of retirement and assisted living facilities. *Courtesy of Valley Care Association.*

On December 28, 1981, Aleppo Township revised the zoning ordinance to allow construction of the nursing home as a conditional use.

In May 1982, the board exercised its option to purchase the property. The sewage agreement with Aleppo Township was completed in October, and the Aleppo property was purchased on November 10 for $250,000. The board pushed to have working drawings completed promptly so that construction could begin as soon as possible.

To meet Federal Housing Administration requirements, the board voted to form a wholly owned subsidiary corporation to own and operate the nursing home, which was to be named Valley Care Nursing Home Incorporated. The people who served on the board of VCA would also be officers and directors of this corporation.

Other significant steps taken in 1982 included:

- Review and approval from the Health Services Agency (which stated that the upper limit of an approvable project would be $35,000 per bed or $4.2 million total cost with 10 percent equity required)
- Receipt of a Certificate of Need from the State Department of Health
- Commitments from Mellon Bank and Pittsburgh National Bank for loans up to $600,000 to guarantee outstanding pledges
- Preparation to officially enter the Social Security system on January 1, 1983

On April 9, 1983, the FHA approved a mortgage, and on April 11, the U.S. Department of Housing and Urban Development approved a bond sale.

GROUND-BREAKING CEREMONY

The ground-breaking ceremony was held on April 10, 1983, and was followed by a reception. The Adult Day Care Center, already operating in the Aleppo Township Municipal Building, was open for tours.

The Reverend Russell W. Turner gave the invocation, with remarks by VCA president Robert Ferguson. The Reverend Jezreel Toliver gave the benediction. Representatives of each of the founding organizations put their shovels to work to dig into the construction site. They were:

- Donald Spalding of SVH
- Marjorie Theys of Friendship House
- Paul D. Ramsey of the Sewickley Senior Citizens Club
- Alice Hays of Union Aid Society
- Reverend George B. Wirth of the Sewickley Ministerium

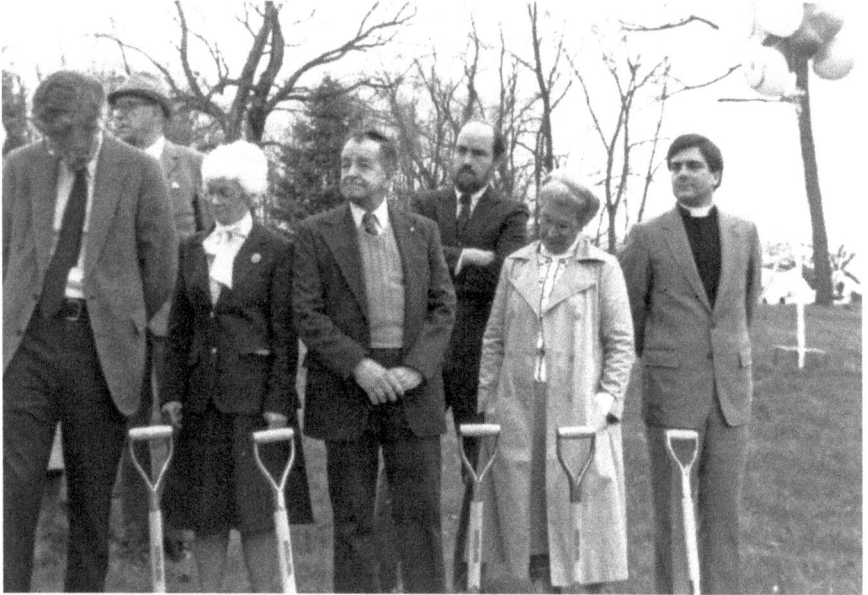

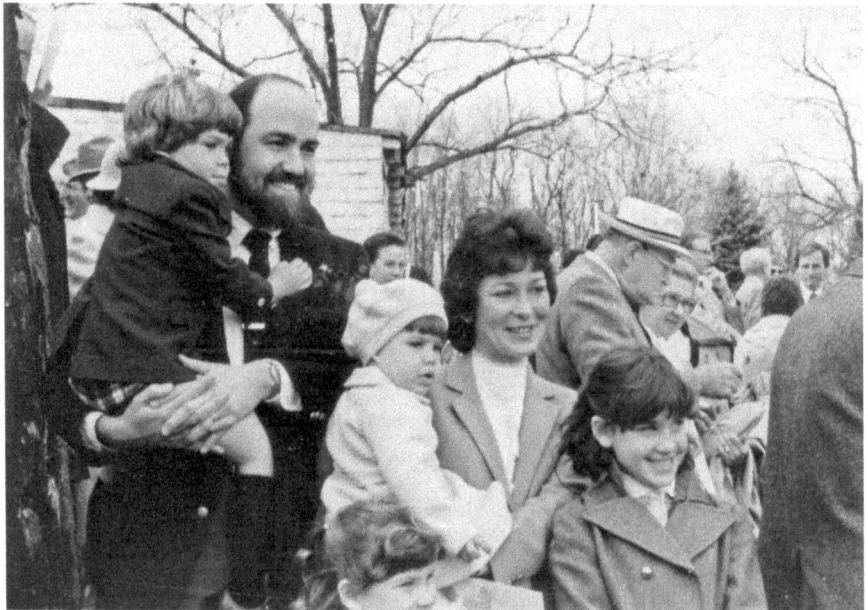

CONSTRUCTION UNDERWAY

Construction began in spring 1983 and moved along rapidly. By late September, construction was 60 percent complete. By the October 1983 annual meeting, the construction of the nursing home was 70 percent complete.

Mellon Stuart Company, general contractor for the nursing home, reported construction costs:

- Materials: $3,351,758.17
- Labor: $108,140.26
- Accounting and consulting services: $3,500.00
- Miscellaneous materials: $916.48

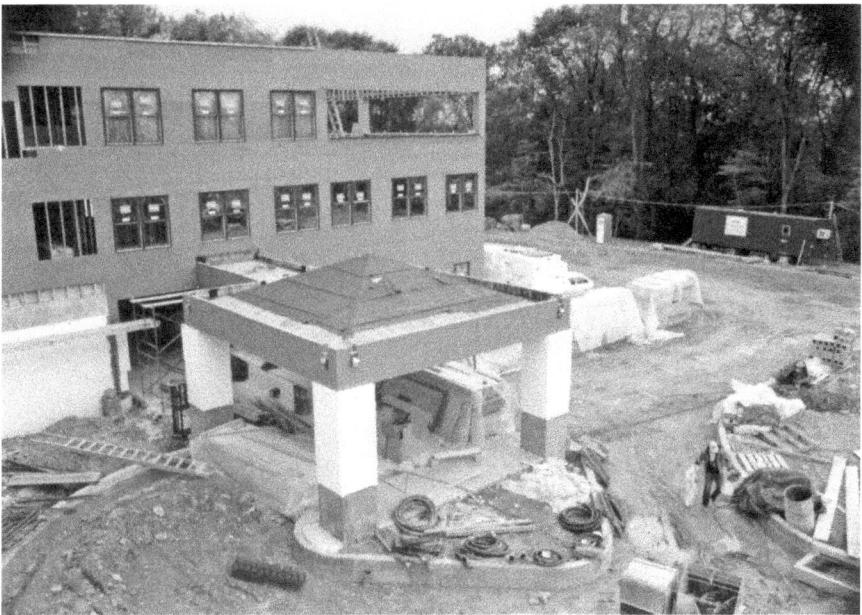

Above: A front view of the covered entrance to Valley Care Nursing Home as it appeared under construction in 1984. *Courtesy of Valley Care Association.*

Opposite, top: Donald Spalding, Marjorie Theys, Paul Ramsey, Alice Hays and Reverend George B. Wirth attend the ground-breaking ceremony on April 10, 1983. *Courtesy of Valley Care Association.*

Opposite, bottom: Dr. Joseph and Mary Jane Bikowski and family attend the ground-breaking ceremony. *Courtesy of Valley Care Association.*

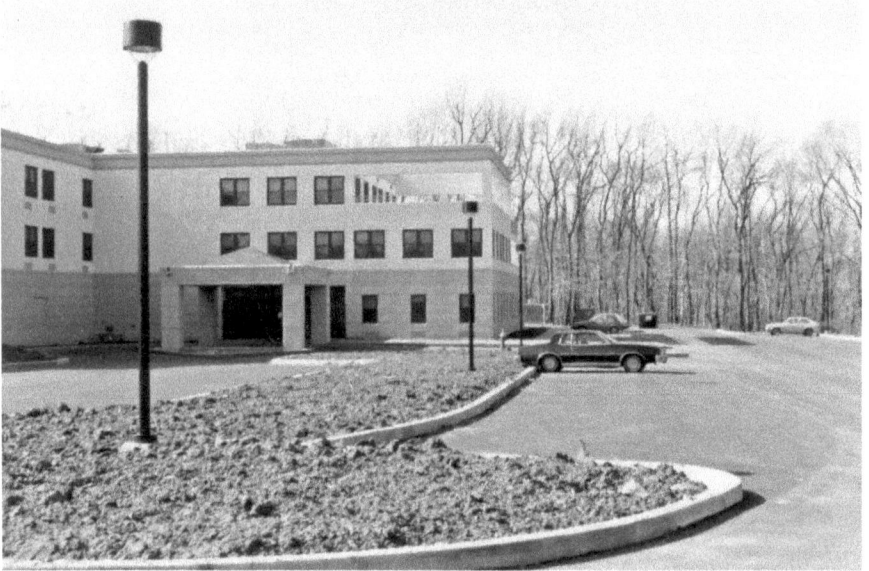

Valley Care Nursing Home's parking lot neared completion in 1984. *Courtesy of Valley Care Association.*

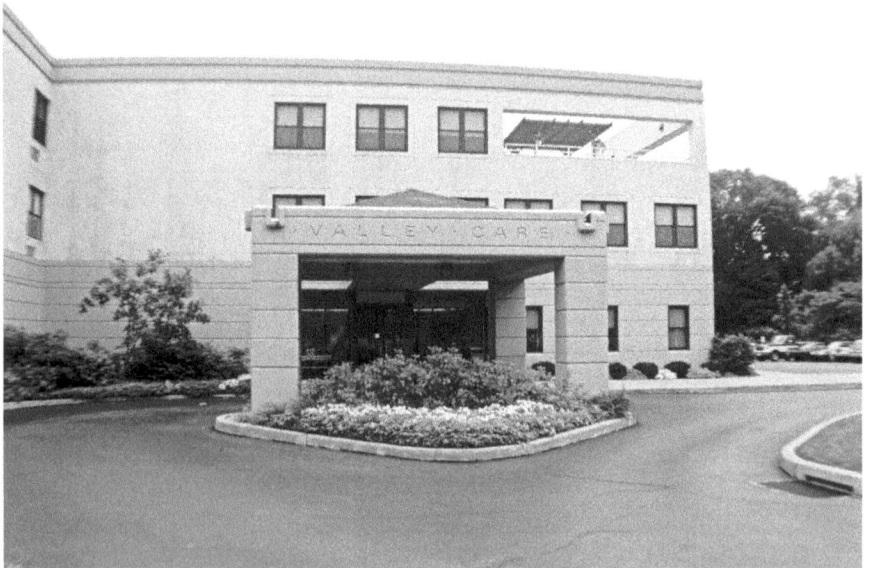

The covered entrance protected visitors to the nursing home from rain and snow. *Courtesy of Ray Geffel.*

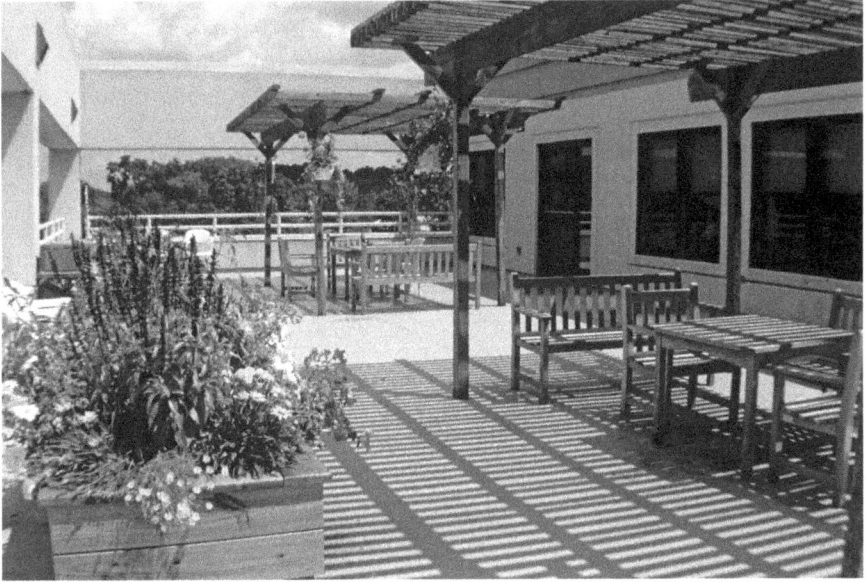

Flowers brighten the décor of the patio at the nursing home in 1992. *Courtesy of Ray Geffel.*

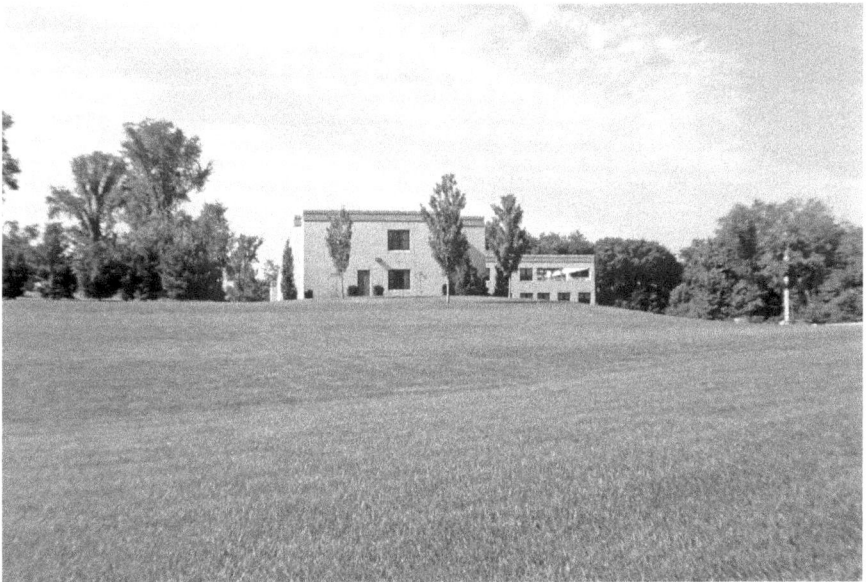

Valley Care Nursing Home was situated on seven of twenty-six acres, leaving space for additional development. *Courtesy of Ray Geffel.*

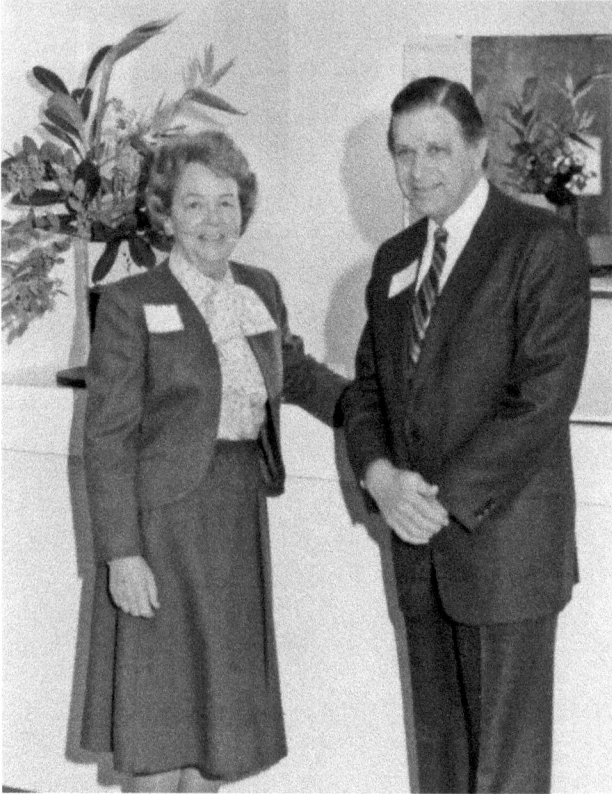

VCA board members Virginia "Deedo" Ramsburg and Marvin Wedeen attend the nursing home open house in 1984. *Courtesy of Valley Care Association.*

When completed, the three-story, concrete building at 1190 Merriman Road had one wing off the main corridor and a portico entrance with a circular driveway. Terraces on each floor allowed residents to enjoy the grand views of the Ohio Valley from the hills of Aleppo Township.

The sixty-three single- and double-occupancy rooms had a total capacity of 120 beds: 88 for patients needing intermediate care and 32 for patients needing skilled care. There was a 22-bed Staunton Unit for Alzheimer's and dementia patients.

Virginia "Deedo" Ramsburg chaired the decorating committee, creating an interior design based on solidarity, security and serenity. "Without Deedo's superb touch, Valley Care Nursing Home would not be the lovely care facility that it is," said Betts Moore.[15] Area residents donated a television, paintings, plants, an aquarium and a piano.

OPEN HOUSE AND GRAND OPENING

When someone is staying at Valley Care, we want them to feel that this is home.
—Judy Comer, first administrator of Valley Care Nursing Home

Valley Care Nursing Home held an open house on March 11, 1984, with more than six hundred people attending. Trustees and staff members conducted tours, showing guests the entire building—from board room to laundry room, including the kitchen, residents' rooms, therapy rooms, shower rooms, the chaplain's office and the airy dining room, which overlooked a terrace and woodsy scene beyond.

The doors of Valley Care Nursing Home opened for its first three residents on March 12, 1984. The initial staff had six registered nurses, but 110 staff members would eventually be needed when the facility reached capacity. This would include registered nurses, practical nurses, nurse's aides, dietary aides and administrators. About 50 percent of the nursing home employees were from the local service area.

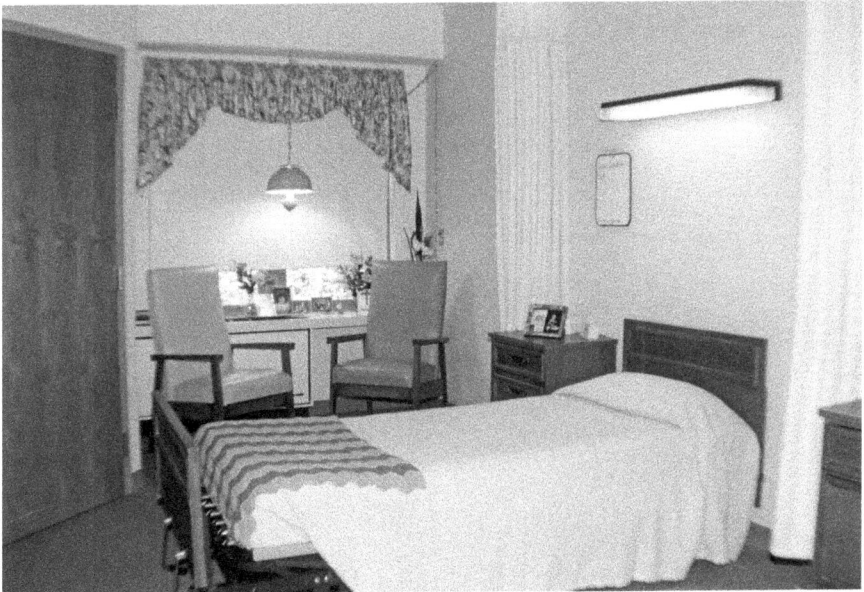

Residents' rooms were bright and comfortable with automatically adjustable beds added in 1992. *Courtesy of Ray Geffel.*

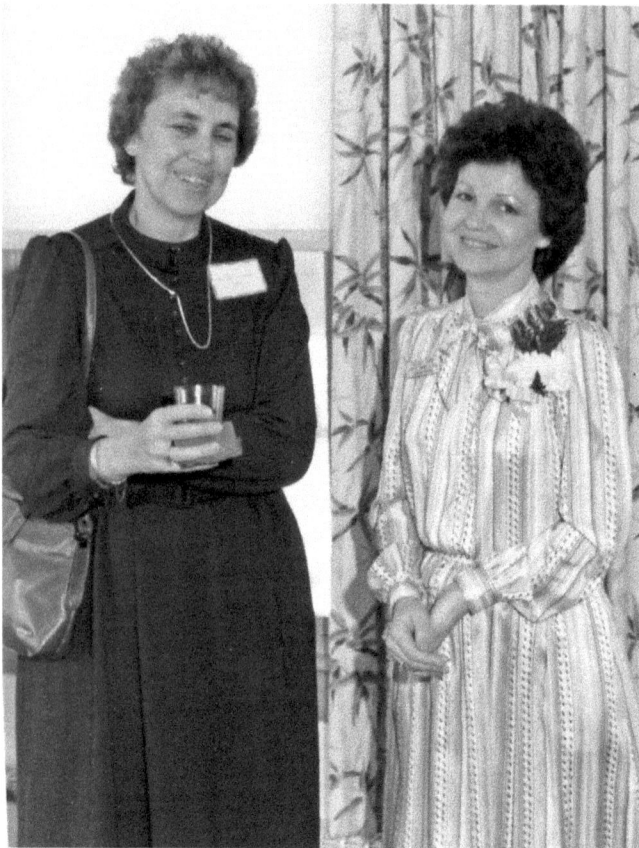

Left: Lannie Gartner, VCA board member (*left*), and Judy Comer, Valley Care Nursing Home administrator, chat at the 1984 nursing home open house. *Courtesy of Valley Care Association.*

Below: Tours of the Valley Care Nursing Home kitchen are held at the open house in 1984. *Courtesy of Valley Care Association.*

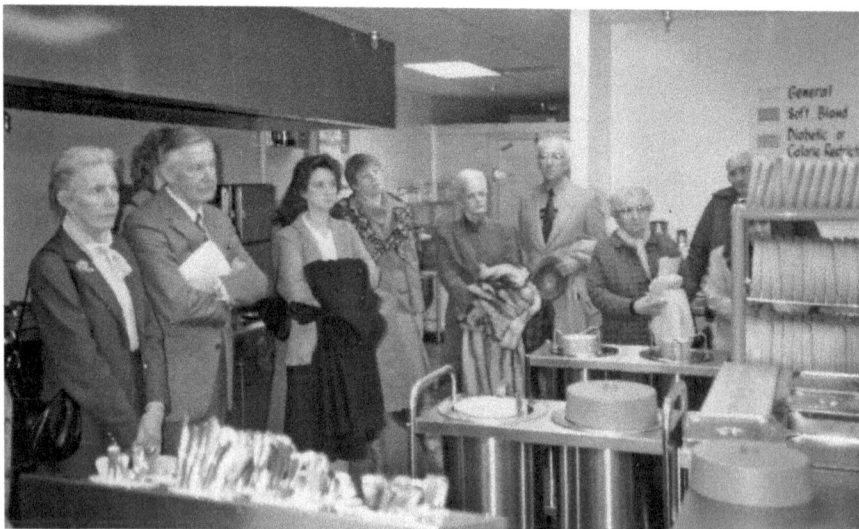

RESIDENT PROFILE: MATTIE RUCKER BRAXTON

Mattie Rucker Braxton celebrated her 100th birthday, on Labor Day, September 3, 1985, in Valley Care Nursing Home. She said, "There were quite a few colored people when I came here, but I guess they're all gone but me. Guess I'm about the only one still hanging around."

Mattie and her husband, Roy, moved to Sewickley in 1907. An active member of the Triumph Baptist Church, she worked for private families—often in Edgeworth. "I was always in the kitchen or the laundry. That's what I liked to do, cook, and wash and iron," she said. Mattie traveled with her employers to their homes at the ocean during the summer.

"I worked hard all my life and got my own—my home and all I need and I want. I was independent." Regarding her secret to her long life, she said, "Take care of your body. Don't you abuse it and don't let anyone else abuse it. Get plenty of rest, and eat the right foods and work hard. Hard work never killed nobody."[*]

* Bettie Cole, *Sewickley Herald*, August 21, 1985.

During the next year, both the staff and the number of residents grew steadily:

- March 30, 1984: 28 full- and part-time employees for 3.6 residents (average occupancy over the month)
- June 30, 1984: 84 employees for 59 residents
- August 30, 1984: 107 employees for 83 residents
- June 1985: 117 employees for 112 residents, or 94 percent of capacity

The eleven attending physicians in various specialties were on the SVH medical staff. Richard Cassoff, MD, an internal medicine specialist from Ambridge, was the medical director.

THE FIRST TWO YEARS

The 1984–85 VCA Annual Report stated that the nursing home was providing a superior quality of care. The staff was alert to residents' needs and suggested changes that could improve their care. The financial results showed that the operation could continue to offer quality care at a reasonable rate.

The first full year of operation was described "by the numbers" in the report:

- 354 people were admitted; 77 recovered to return home
- 50 percent of the residents were on medical assistance; 10 percent were covered by the Medicare program; with the rest on private pay or personal insurance plans
- 70 percent of the residents were female and 30 percent male, with an average age of 77
- Residents received 10,729 physical therapy treatments, 491 occupational therapy treatments and 754 speech therapy treatments
- The activities department provided 2,444 activities, including prescribed activities for non-ambulatory residents

Most of the residents were from Sewickley, Bellevue, Avalon, Ambridge or the Moon/Coraopolis area, with the rest from twenty-six other communities. Residents came to the nursing home through various routes:

- 70 percent were referred from hospitals, mostly from SVH, along with eighteen other hospitals
- 17 percent were admitted directly from a family home
- 13 percent came from other nursing homes or care facilities

During the course of the year, the nursing home added equipment, services, activities and quality training for employees. They also hired new specialists, such as a chaplain, art therapist and music therapist.

The nursing home had a resident council, a representative body of residents who met monthly to plan activities and share mutual interests and concerns. The group represented the residents and conveyed their concerns to administration and the board. Activities included small fund-raisers, such as producing and selling a cookbook.

In July 1985, Mary Mathews, who was now working as director of social services and admissions, and Karen Kopco Davis, activities director, started a family support group to help residents' family members deal with having a loved one in a nursing home. The group met monthly to discuss issues, such as making visits count, handling sensory losses in the elderly, adjusting to a nursing home, feeling guilty and reversing roles.

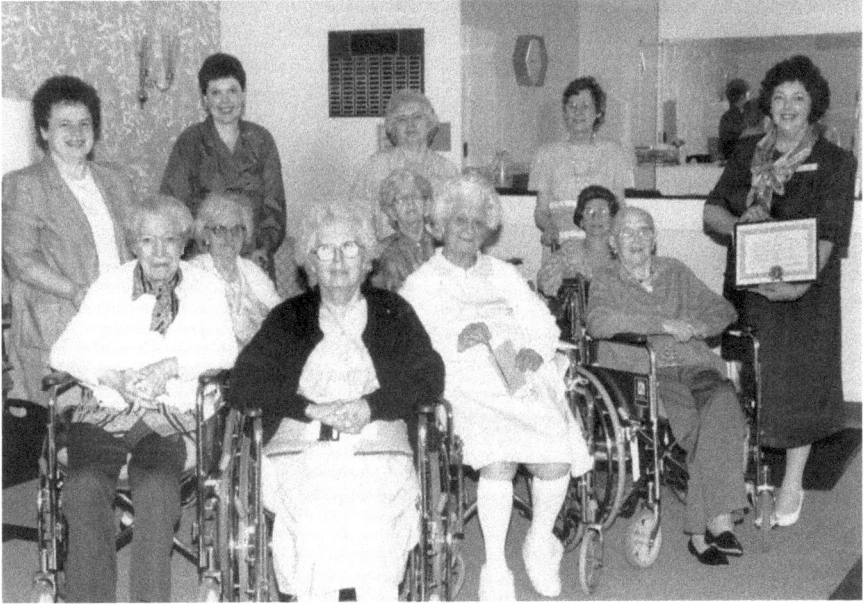

The Resident Council of Valley Care Nursing Home meets in 1985 to discuss concerns with administration. *Courtesy of Stanley Briller.*

In 1985, VCA purchased nineteen additional acres adjacent to the nursing home for $190,000, giving it a total of forty-five acres in Aleppo Township.

In winter 1986, the nursing home was awarded a three-year Certificate of Accreditation by the Joint Commission on Accreditation of Hospitals. This certification required a rigorous onsite evaluation, confirming that the nursing home met high standards of quality patient care and safety.

SPECIAL EVENTS AND RECREATIONAL ACTIVITIES

Special events helped nursing home residents connect with the traditions of their past while keeping their minds and bodies alert and active. The holiday dinner started in 1986 and became an annual event. Families joined their loved ones at this special dinner, and all were served by staff, the board of trustees and community volunteers who wore candy-striped aprons. Young boys and girls greeted the families as they arrived and passed out candy canes.

"You always went to Grandmother's house for the holiday dinner. She was the official hostess then, and she still is here at Valley Care," said Diane

---

RESIDENT PROFILE: THOMAS

"Last year one of our parishioners, Thomas, was a patient at Valley Care [Nursing Home]. Thom suffered from AIDS and died at Valley Care. [We] were impressed by the care and concern of the staff at Valley Care for Thom. Thom himself, on one occasion, expressed to me how pleased he was with his care. I visited him there several times and always found that he was clean and well cared for. The nursing staff was sensitive to his condition and treated him with dignity. As you know, this is not always the case with AIDS patients. Diane Martinez [nursing home administrator], in particular, and also the nurses, assistants, etc. are to be commended for their professional approach."

—*Harry E. Nichols, pastor of Saint Veronica Church in Ambridge,*
in a 1991 letter to Valley Care President James Alexander

Martinez, nursing home administrator. "When I see family members interacting with the residents, it gives me such good feelings."

Along with holiday decorations there would be Christmas carols played on the piano. "The arrival of grandchildren brings such joy to the residents," said Mathews. "This is truly an intergenerational celebration."

But the fun didn't stop with Christmas. In addition to monthly birthday parties, other holidays were special occasions, with staff and residents dressing up, making decorations or throwing parties. These activities kept the residents feeling like part of the larger community in their home away from home.

Educational programming covered topics such as healthy eating and the expansion of the Pittsburgh International Airport. Recreational activities rounded out the calendar with cooking, baking, sewing, horticulture, art and ceramics, as well as trips to a flower show, an aviary and baseball games.

VCA was given a 1985 AMC Eagle station wagon, which staff members used to take residents to the dentist; to swimming therapy at the Sewickley YMCA; and on field trips to the Pittsburgh Zoo, parks, shopping and restaurants. The nursing home even participated in the Sewickley Memorial Day Parade, with some residents riding in a convertible. In April 1985, VCA purchased a seven-passenger van for the nursing home to help with these transportation needs.

In 1986, with two pianos on the premises, the nursing home welcomed performers from schools and churches to entertain the residents. In July

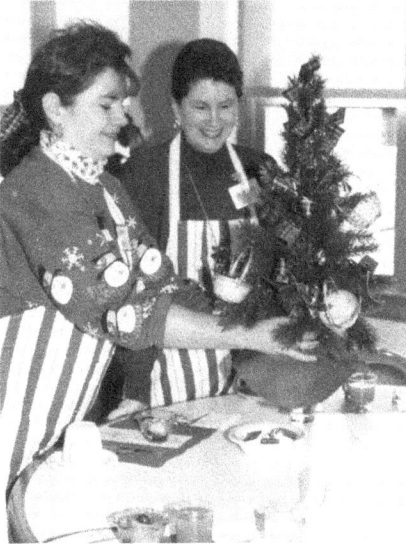

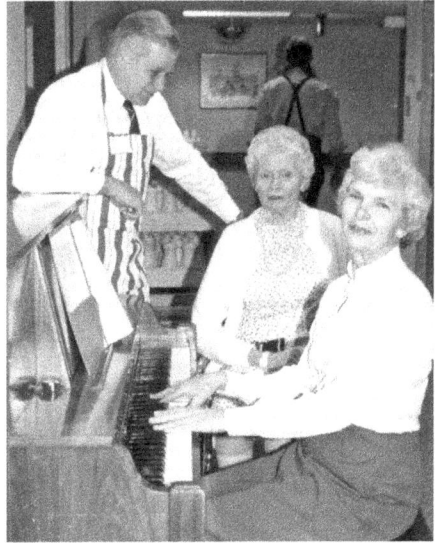

Left: Lynn Harvey, director of housekeeping and laundry, and Mary Mathews, director of admissions and social services, prepare Christmas decorations in 1993. *Courtesy of Valley Care Association.*

Right: Board president Marvin Wedeen sings carols with nursing home resident Virginia Perin and pianist Ann Cahouet during the holiday dinner. *Courtesy of Valley Care Association.*

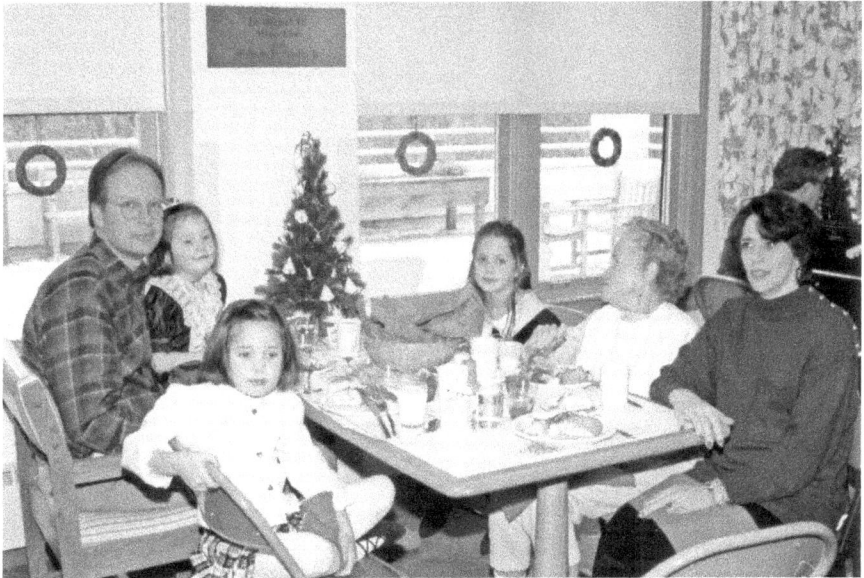

The nursing home holiday party in 1995 allowed the whole family to join Grandma for Christmas dinner. *Courtesy of Valley Care Association.*

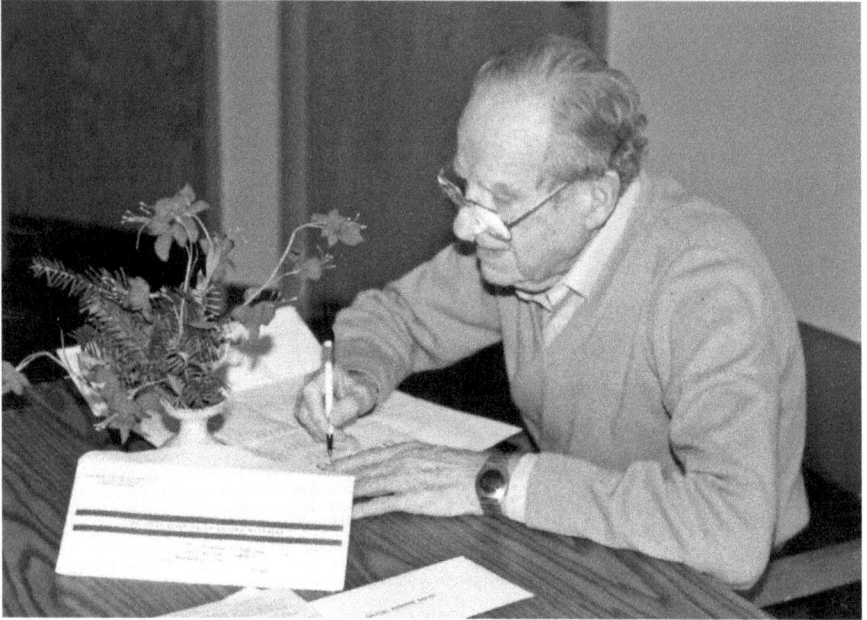

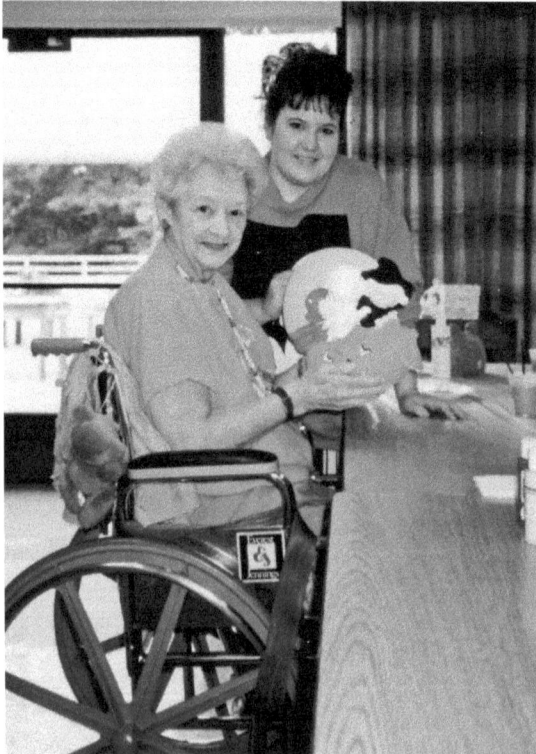

Above: Nursing home residents vote in the presidential election in 1984. *Courtesy of Valley Care Association.*

Left: Nursing home resident Laurentine Hollopeter tries her hand at ceramics with Michele Scholdel, art instructor, 1994. *Courtesy of Valley Care Association.*

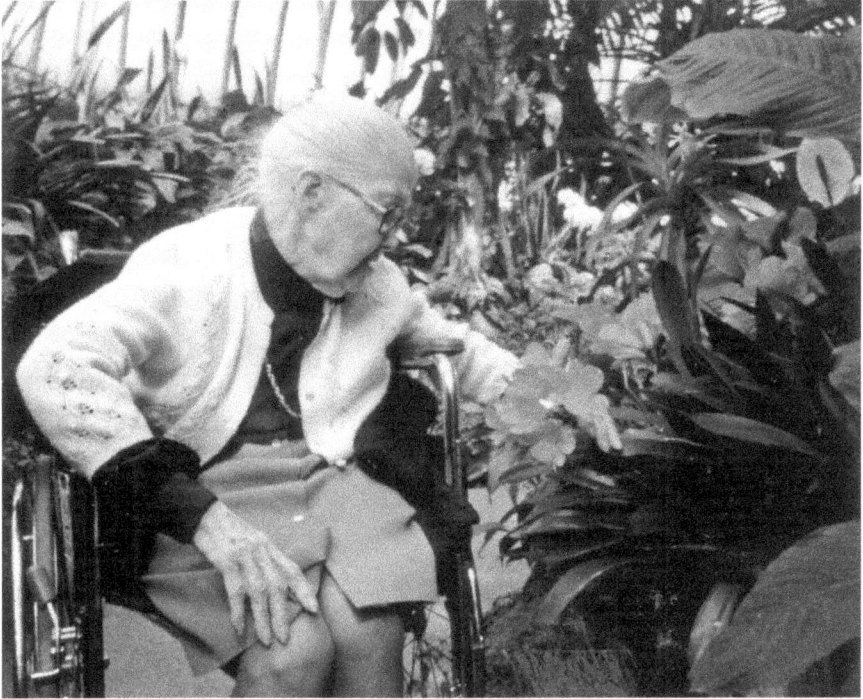

Elizabeth Roberts, Valley Care Nursing Home resident, takes time to smell the flowers on a trip to Phipps Conservatory in 1992. *Courtesy of Valley Care Association.*

1987, sixteen children from Saint James Bible School in Sewickley came to sing and play musical instruments.

The Valley Care chorus of twenty residents gathered once a week to sing and socialize. Sing-alongs were also popular, with music time being a favorite activity. Residents who had suffered strokes and couldn't talk were sometimes able to sing, according to Karen Davis, music therapist.

> *This was a Cadillac operation that was being supported by a bicycle revenue stream. Having the Resident Council, comprehensive dementia services, a family support group, special events, holiday dinners…all spoke of the idealism and compassion that prevailed and allowed the original mission to flow into the care and life of every patient and family.*
> *—Dan Brooks, MD, VCE board member*

RESIDENT PROFILE: CHRISTINA BRADLEY

Christina was a local caterer for forty-five years, starting her vocation as a volunteer cook during World War II. She and other women of the Presbyterian Church of Sewickley prepared evening meals six days a week for army and navy personnel stationed nearby.

At age eighty-one, while living at Valley Care Nursing Home, Bradley retained an active mind and the *joie de vivre* of a much younger woman. She regularly attended poetry hour and Bible study. On one outing to Osborne Elementary School for National Days, her two great-granddaughters, Monica Humbles, six, and Joy Humbles, nine, served her English tea.

For the *Care Connection*, the nursing home's monthly newsletter, she wrote, "I now use a wheelchair. Often when I sit in the third floor lounge watching the chairs come in for lunch or dinner, each occupant brings with them something to admire—like the quiet patience as they wait for their trays. The loving aides or nurses feed them. Many pass by the dining room and give a cheery hello or mention something about a ball game or a word about the important issues of the day. Those who are able to walk about come to sit and talk with me. No matter whether on foot or wheelchair, they are beautiful people."

SPIRITUAL COUNSELING

In January 1983, VCA's pastoral care committee recommended that the nursing home plan for a part-time chaplain to conduct church services and serve the spiritual needs of the residents. The pastoral care committee submitted seven proposals to foundations to fund the chaplaincy program. These were unsuccessful, and in 1984, VCA contributed $7,500 to support the program for the first year.

In 1984 and 1985, Reverend Russell Turner conducted spiritual services at the nursing home. He also trained lay volunteers to be chaplain's assistants, visiting residents, listening to their concerns and giving guidance. Two students from the Trinity School of Ministry in Ambridge also came to the nursing home for ten hours each week to assist with pastoral duties. Reverend J.S. Meenan brought communion to the Catholic residents from 1984 until his resignation in 1988.

Turner retired in the fall of 1985, and the Reverend Jean-Jacques D'Aoust, PhD, assistant rector of Fox Chapel Episcopal Church, became part-time chaplain at the nursing home.

He was eventually succeeded by the Reverend Bruce Bryce, who served from 1988 to 1991, for about ten hours each week. Bryce was described in the VCA newsletter as an "affable, ecumenically minded minister ready to meet the spiritual needs of the community." Bryce was the full-time chaplain at SVH and considered Valley Care Nursing Home an extension of his hospital ministry, since many patients became residents there.

Later, Bryce wrote a column for the VCA newsletter. In the summer 1992 issue he wrote:

> *I am here to serve the residents, not to lead them. It's my job to release the internal feelings about their individual concepts of God by using their lifelong religious teachings and customs…the ones they have had for seven, eight, or nine decades.*
>
> *Each one of them faces eternity. They have few requirements beyond basic personal comfort. They want dignity. They want a realization that they are important to someone. By developing spirituality, they can still mature and realize that their God is genuine and personal.*

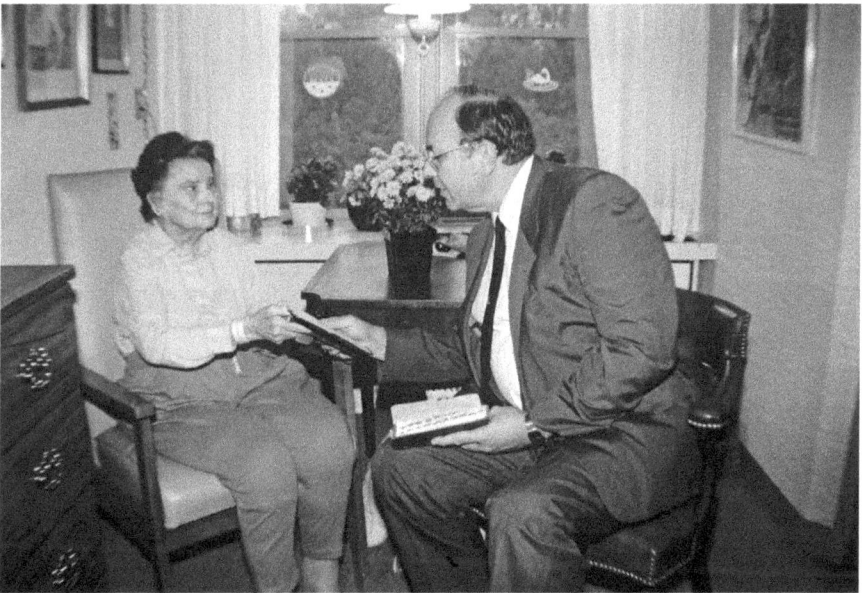

Reverend Bruce Bryce reads the Bible with a resident. Bryce served as chaplain at the Valley Care Nursing Home from 1988 to 1991. *Courtesy of Valley Care Association.*

SPECIAL CARE FOR DEMENTIA PATIENTS

Nowhere at Valley Care is the concept of community more vividly or meaningfully demonstrated than in the Staunton Wing.
—J. Robert Ferguson Jr., in a report to Staunton Farm Foundation

In 1980, Alzheimer's affected at least 2 million Americans and was the fourth leading cause of death among the elderly. Alzheimer's was the most common cause of dementia among older adults. Of the 1.3 million elderly Americans in nursing homes, it was estimated that 300,000 had Alzheimer's. Despite the prevalence of this disease, in 1985 only about one hundred nursing homes offered proper treatment.[16]

VCA was ahead of the curve in its approach to patients with mental difficulties. The board designated twenty-two beds in a separate wing of the nursing home for patients who "are mentally impaired, have Alzheimer's, or other dementia." This special unit was named the Staunton Wing in recognition of a $525,000 contribution from the Staunton Farm Foundation.

According to Valley Care Nursing Home administrator Judy Comer, research into Alzheimer's shows that the more attention and activity a

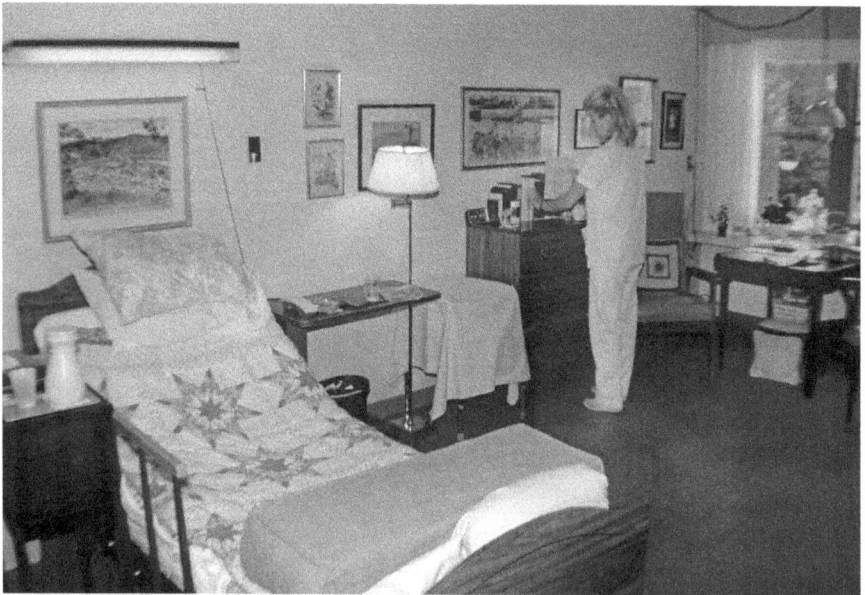

Residents brought many personal items to decorate their rooms at the nursing home. *Courtesy of Ray Geffel.*

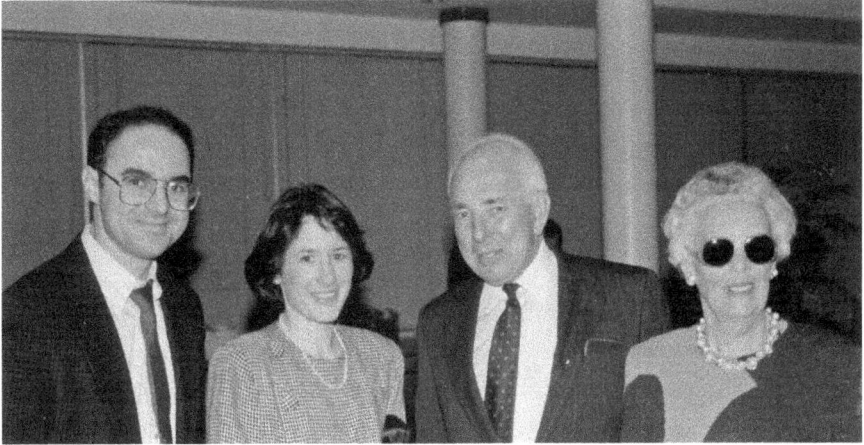

Dr. Chris O'Donnell, nursing home medical director, and his wife, Jean, at a VCA annual meeting with board president James Alexander and his wife, Helen. *Courtesy of Valley Care Association.*

disoriented person receives, the more stable they become.[17] Nurses and therapists, along with security, housekeeping and maintenance staff, were trained by the psychiatric teams of SVH's Staunton Clinic on the special needs of elderly patients experiencing psychiatric difficulties. Clinical staff had a twenty-day training rotation in the psychiatric units of the hospital and the nursing home.

While the state required 2.5 hours of direct nursing care per patient, Valley Care Nursing Home provided 3.5 hours in the nursing home and 4.9 hours in the Staunton Wing.

Rocking chairs in the Staunton Wing lounge areas helped residents relax. The unit also included plenty of space for people to walk around, including a fenced-in outdoor area with edible plants. Patient rooms were decorated with the residents' own furniture, stuffed animals and other personal mementos to help them feel at home.

Valley Care provided dementia patients with Wander Guard bracelets, which had sensors that tripped an alarm if a patient opened a door to leave. "Patients with Alzheimer's tend to wander a lot and have behavioral problems," said Dr. Chris O'Donnell, one of Valley Care Nursing Home's medical directors. "If we can get them active with daily walks, we can reduce their propensity to wander."

Special Attention and Loving Care

The Staunton Clinic staff provided reality orientation and sensory stimulation, in addition to physical and activity therapy. Some of the activities were art and music therapy, exercise, word search games, flash cards and puzzles. All senses were used to redevelop mental stimulus.

"We were on the cutting edge in Alzheimer's care," said Mathews. "There were many challenges that the social services and staff had to deal with.

"We used to give residents and Adult Day Care clients with Alzheimer's 'reality orientation,' stressing the date, the weather, and the next holiday to try to ground them in reality. This was mandated by the state. Years later the philosophy was to have the caregivers meet the residents where they were, on their level, in their reality," she said.

Initially, the goal was to provide the care necessary to keep a resident healthy and comfortable, according to Mathews. "As the years passed, the nursing home adopted a different philosophy of care, and staff strived to keep each resident as independent and capable as they could be," she said.

The residents were free to set their own pace within limited control. They were not overly medicated or restrained in their beds. Several women chose not to go to sleep until four o'clock in the morning, an arrangement that the staff accommodated.

Nurses and aides were specially selected to provide not only the right physical care but also the love and reassurance these patients needed. Caring for older people who could not remember instructions from one day to the next was a lot like caring for a toddler.

In a 1985 report to Staunton Farm Foundation, administrators shared the results of the first year of operation, with forty-four admissions to the Staunton Wing, stating, "At Valley Care we attempt to help residents rebuild their lost communities. Although families come and bring grandchildren and sometimes even the family pet, after the visit is over the resident is left to his own resources again. Nowhere at Valley Care is the concept of community more vividly or meaningfully demonstrated than in the Staunton Wing. Because of the residents' decreased cognitive abilities…it is important to emphasize the emotional aspects of their existence."

Some residents required psychiatric help upon admission to Valley Care Nursing Home, but they improved with treatment. Ferguson stated that in 1984–85, six residents rehabilitated and returned home, while six were moved to another area of the nursing home due to an increase in alertness. "One rehabilitated resident who returned to his home is now seen at Valley Care visiting his father," he said.

SATISFIED FAMILIES

Several family members wrote letters expressing their satisfaction with the care at the Staunton Clinic. Mr. and Mrs. James Morris wrote, "My husband and I were up to visit his mother, Alberta Morris, and each time we visit her, we know we made the right choice by placing her at Valley Care. We had her out for a short walk on the grounds but she was most anxious to get back. We were so taken by her friends welcoming her back. We know now that she has made this her home and is very happy and secure with her friends and surroundings....She was like a little girl, telling us about her friend fixing her nails and putting on makeup. It is these little extras that keep her happy. I know the nurses do not have to do these things, but they are loved for it."

Another family member wrote, "I am very contented that my little Mom, Ethel Durgan, is in Staunton Wing. She knows her name now, and has someone to talk to. And she's kept very, very clean, and they even put her hair up, and she loves the food. Everyone raps nursing homes but this one is okay in my eyes."

4

Maintaining Top-Quality Care, 1984–96

D iane Martinez left an administrative position at a seven-hundred-bed nursing home in Johnstown, Pennsylvania, to become administrator of the Valley Care Nursing Home, serving from 1986 to 1992. Her first nursing position was in obstetrics, dealing with the labor and delivery of babies, so, as she said, "I have gone through the life cycle in my career."

"Here you know the residents by name, know their families and the employees. This is a people business, and I like to know the people I am working with and the people we are caring for....These people become a part of you. You get attached, and sometimes it's hard when they die or they get better and can go home. Either way, it's hard to say goodbye," said Martinez.[18]

In the summer of 1989, as the nursing home celebrated its fifth anniversary, an addition to the Staunton Wing was under construction. The additional space provided better services and security, adding eight beds, a nursing station, a dining room and a recreation room. The cost was $550,000, with $250,000 contributed by VCA and the rest from charitable donations.

On May 23, 1990, during National Nursing Home Week, Sewickley mayor William H. Colbert issued a proclamation urging all citizens to "take pride in caring by visiting Valley Care Nursing Home and lending support to the residents, staff and volunteers who make long-term care something for which this community truly can be proud."

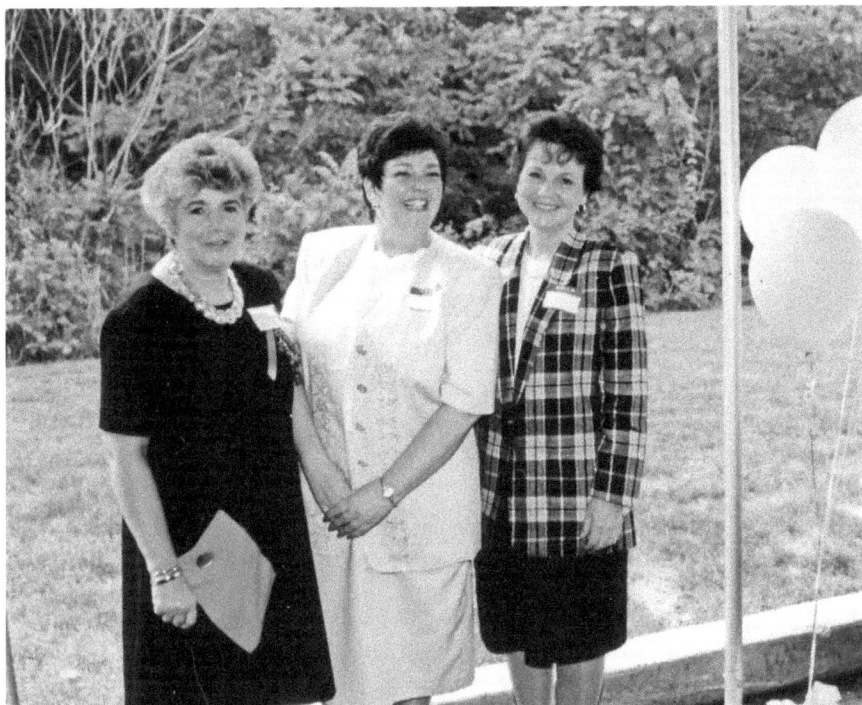

Three nursing home administrators, B.J. Franks, Diane Martinez and Judy Comer, reunite at the tenth anniversary party in 1994. *Courtesy of Valley Care Association.*

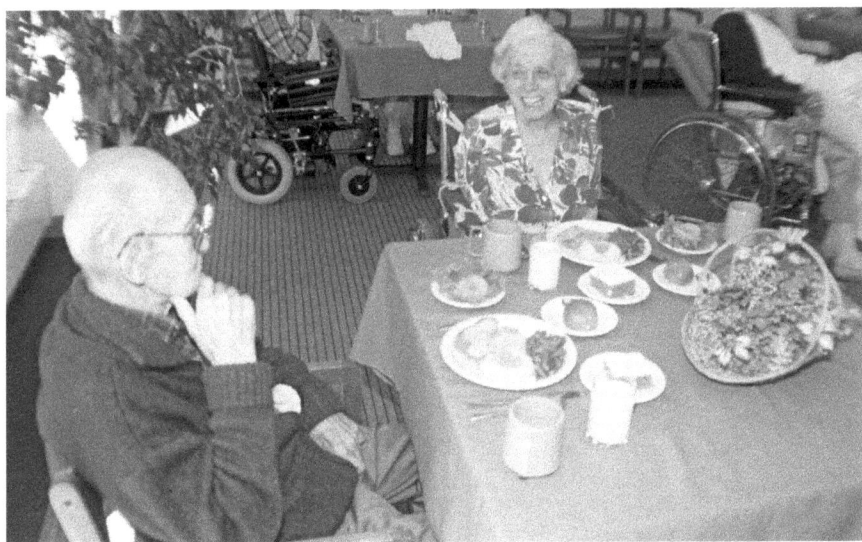

Mealtime was always a special occasion in the nursing home dining room. *Courtesy of Ray Geffel.*

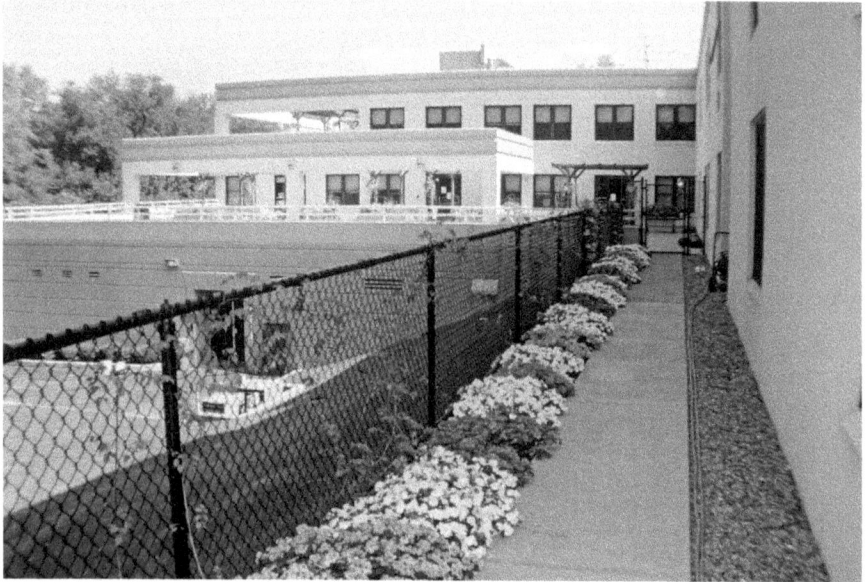

The walkway along the side of the nursing home that led to the patio was lined with flowers in the spring of 1992. *Courtesy of Ray Geffel.*

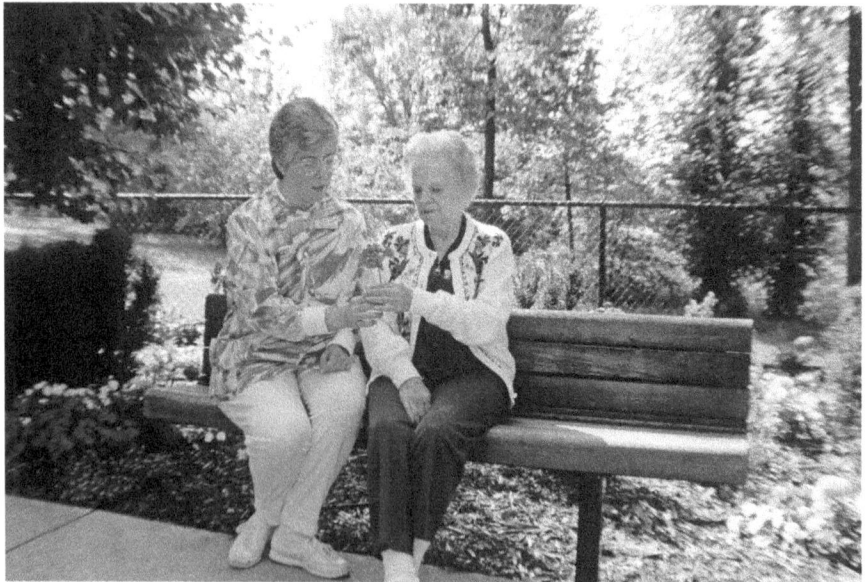

A nurse and resident enjoy the outdoor patio off the Staunton Wing in 1992. *Courtesy of Ray Geffel.*

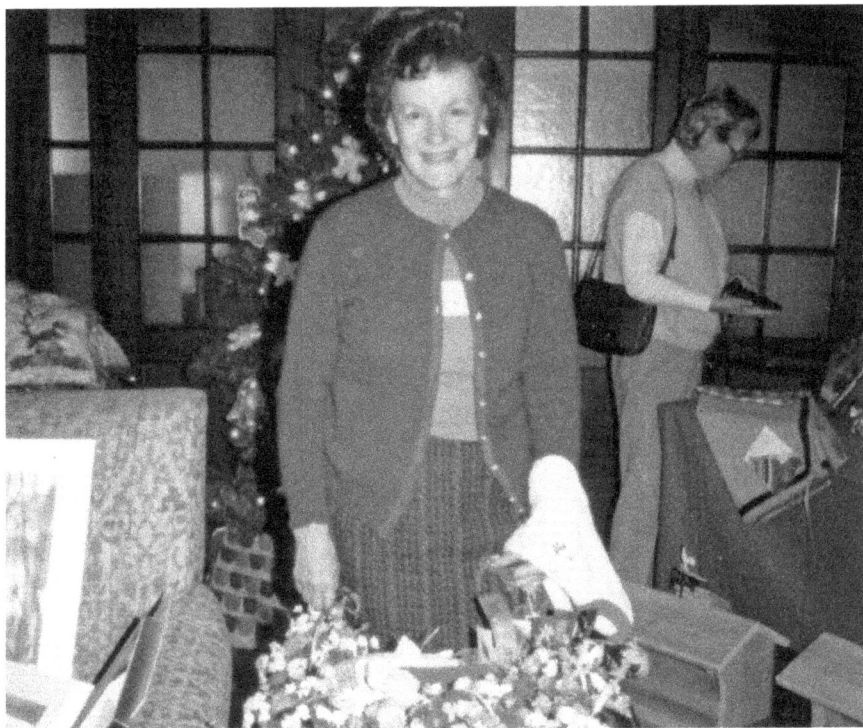

Above: Gwen Ogle, VCA auxiliary and board member and volunteer. *Courtesy of Valley Care Association.*

Right: Sandy Doughty, director of nursing, helps Elizabeth E. Walter, nursing home resident, with a craft project in 1994. *Courtesy of Valley Care Association.*

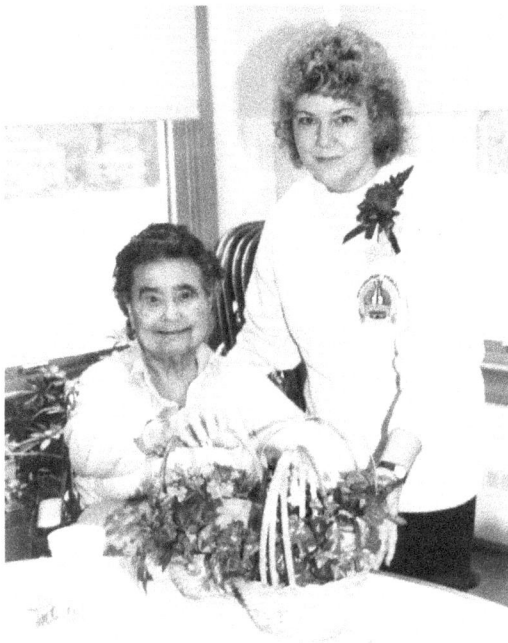

Gwen Ogle, a VCA board member for seventeen years and former president of the Valley Care Auxiliary, said about the nursing home:

Valley Care probably was the best nursing home I've ever seen. And it wasn't because I was on the board. It was because of the mission and the way they cared. The aides always seemed to like what they were doing, and they liked the people. The staff had a good sense of humor. That was the way the residents were treated, with respect and humor. I always had a good feeling about it. I had my mother-in-law there, and I had no complaints.

MARKETING AND FINANCES

Marketing efforts in these years included an ad campaign that Gloria Berry, VCA marketing consultant, worked on with a Pittsburgh ad agency. They came up with a memorable slogan: "We serve 100 grandmothers dinner every night. We spread a lot of love around."

In 1990–91 the daily cost for skilled care at Valley Care Nursing Home was:

- $110 for a semi-private room
- $125 for a private room
- $110 for a semi-private room, Staunton Wing

In comparison, in 2019, the daily costs for the Sturgeon Healthcare Center (the nursing home at Masonic Village) were:

- $387 for a private room
- $376 for a private room with a shared bath

However, the 2019 cost was different for Masonic Village residents who transitioned from independent living to the nursing home. They continued to pay the base monthly fee they paid while living independently, about a third of the price mentioned above.

The nursing home's finances were challenged in 1990–91. This was a result of Pennsylvania delaying adoption of the state budget and Medical Assistance bills going unpaid for six months, costs incurred to stay in compliance with new quality and service standards required by regulatory agencies and Medicaid per diem rates continuing to be inadequate related to actual costs. In addition, Medicare and Blue Cross were unable to agree on who was

Valley Care Nursing Home ran an ad focused on its service to its residents in 1991. *Courtesy of Valley Care Association.*

responsible for payments to nursing homes, halting $100,000 in payments to Valley Care Nursing Home. The 365-day coverage for skilled care under Blue Cross was also discontinued, causing many to lose their insurance coverage. Some converted to Medical Assistance (later called Medicaid).

A 1.8-acre piece of property adjacent to the nursing home became available in 1991. With financial help from local Sewickley foundations, the board purchased the land. VCA now owned a total of forty-seven acres—more than enough land for future expansion of the facility.

RETAINING NURSES AND AIDES

Care for the elderly required continual hiring and training of capable staff to provide the highest quality and experience. From 1990 until 1992, the nursing home was training and hiring an average of thirty-five nurse's aides a year, with turnover at more than 75 percent. Outside staffing agencies were used to support the in-house nursing staff, an arrangement that neither engendered loyalty nor developed a skilled staff.

In 1992, the nursing home began an effort to reduce turnover, using an approach that emphasized teamwork, as recommended by industry studies.

THE BLIZZARD OF 1993

The blizzard that blanketed Pittsburgh on March 13, 1993, was one of a kind. "This is the most snow that ever fell in one day, from midnight to midnight—23.6 inches of snow," said KDKA television meteorologist Dennis Bowman. "You were discouraged from going anywhere, though some people tried to get out and about."

Governor Robert P. Casey declared a state of emergency throughout Pennsylvania. At the Valley Care Nursing Home, many of the staff took on extra shifts to cover for workers who couldn't travel.

"I want to thank you for the tremendous effort you made during the blizzard of '93 to keep Valley Care operational," wrote VCA president James Alexander in a letter. "I know this was not easy and I greatly appreciate the dedication of all who put in long hours over this winter weekend. Be assured that this effort was appreciated not only by me but the whole board and the residents as well."

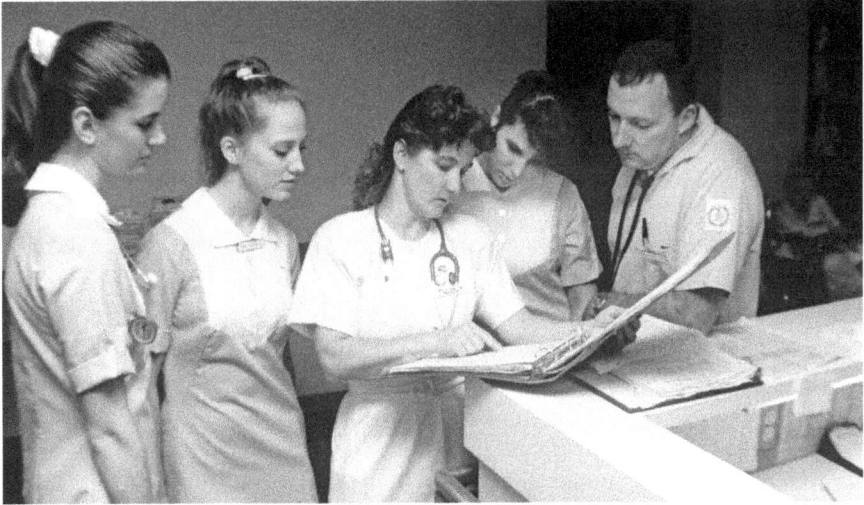

Student nurses gained valuable experience and contributed to residents' care. *Courtesy of Ray Geffel.*

The board brought in a management consulting firm and reorganized personnel, appointing a clinical coordinator for each of the nursing units. Teams were created to cover shifts throughout all twenty-four hours of the day. "Employees now feel they have more input into the operation and are willing to take on more responsibility," stated the 1992 VCA annual report.

In 1992, Peggy Wetzel, director of staff development and quality assurance, directed the VCA state-certified nurse's aide training program of 160 hours in gerontology, anatomy, physiology, geriatrics and gerontics. Continuing education covered such topics as breathing assessment, tracheostomy care, body mechanics and alternatives to psychotropic medications.

Nurse's aides performed demanding, repetitive work for less compensation than the nurses, yet their devotion to caring for very dependent patients was equally important.

During the 1996 fiscal year, the nursing home embarked on a total quality management program, training the entire staff on several initiatives for improvement. As a result, Valley Care Nursing Home achieved the following:

- Decreased use of restraints, while ensuring safety from falls (only 10 of 127 residents needed restraints)
- Improved wound and skin care management

- Expanded physical and occupational therapy efforts
- Expanded restorative nursing and speech pathology programs
- A dramatic 20 percent increase in discharges to home over the prior year

Professional staff were supplemented over the years by nursing, physical therapy and occupational therapy students, who worked at the nursing home to gain real-life experience to augment their studies. As they gained this experience, the nursing home was infused with new ideas, methods and enthusiasm from the students.

CELEBRATING THE TENTH ANNIVERSARY

VCA celebrated the nursing home's tenth anniversary in 1994 with a weekend of activities that included an antique car show, parties and picnics. Mary Mathews and VCA trustee Deedo Ramsburg designed and produced a commemorative flag.

The antique car show included sixty cars, car rides, photo ops, a high-wheel bicycle parade and a raffle. It ran from 10:00 a.m. to 3:00 p.m. on July 30, 1994, on Broad Street in Sewickley. The two-dollar admission fee went to support

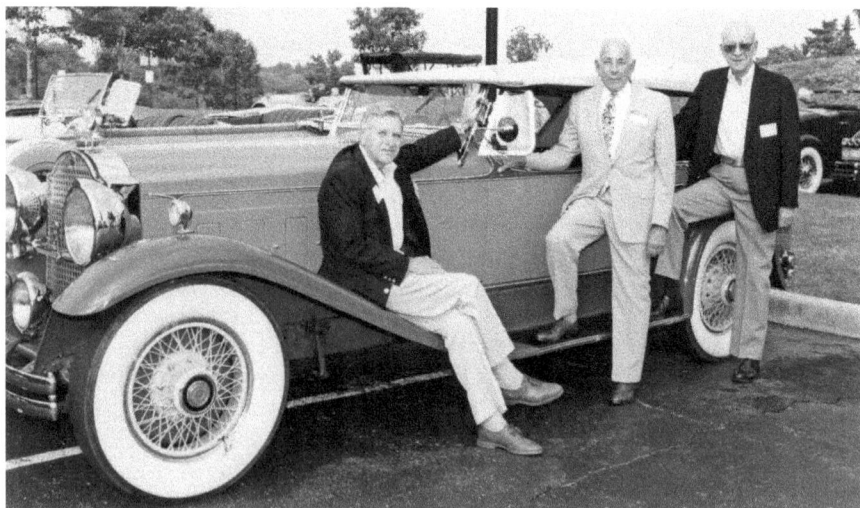

VCA president Marvin Wedeen and past presidents Jim Alexander and Bob Ferguson Jr., pose with a 1930 Packard at the anniversary party in 1994. *Courtesy of Valley Care Association.*

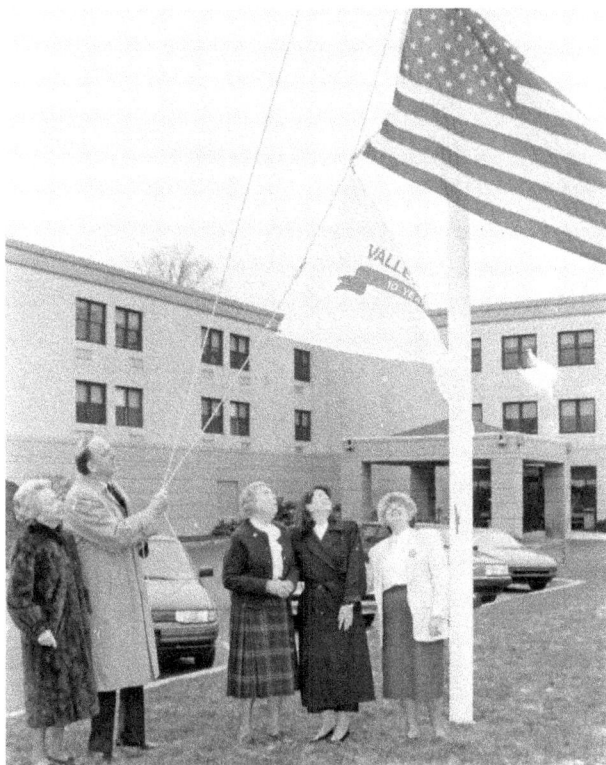

Left: Anniversary committee members Deedo Ramsburg, G. Whitney Snyder, Betty Colbert, Mary Mathews and B.J. Franks raise the flag at the tenth anniversary celebration. *Courtesy of Valley Care Association.*

Below: G. Whitney Snyder drives his 1910 Pierce with Sandy Doughty, director of nursing, and Agatha Moder and Harry Petri, nursing home residents, riding along. *Courtesy of Valley Care Association.*

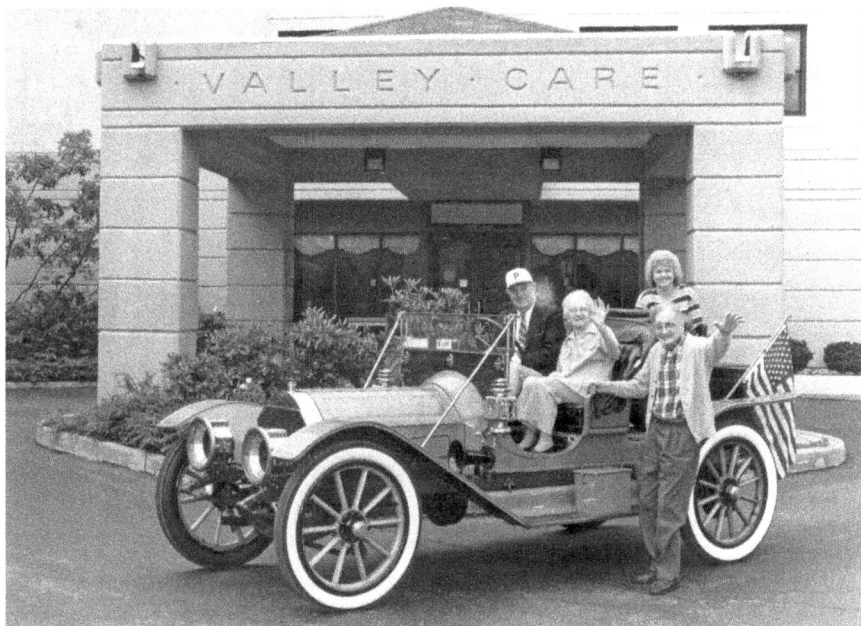

IT'S COMING!...

THE SEWICKLEY ANTIQUE CAR SHOW

60 GREAT CARS

Saturday, July 30
10 a.m. ☞ 3:30 p.m.
Broad Street
Sewickley, Pennsylvania

Admission: **Adults** ONLY **$2** ✱ children (12 & under) **FREE**

RAFFLE! 1979 Mercedes Benz 300TD
Station Wagon ✱ Rides in Antique Cars ✱
For Kids of All Ages ✱ "Old Time" Family Photos

FREE PARKING

Sponsored by
The Transportation & Technology Museum

Proceeds Benefit
Valley Care Nursing Home

For information ✆
(412) 741-1400

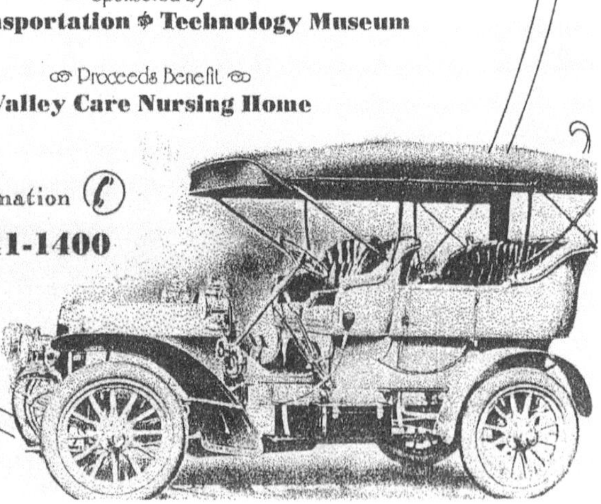

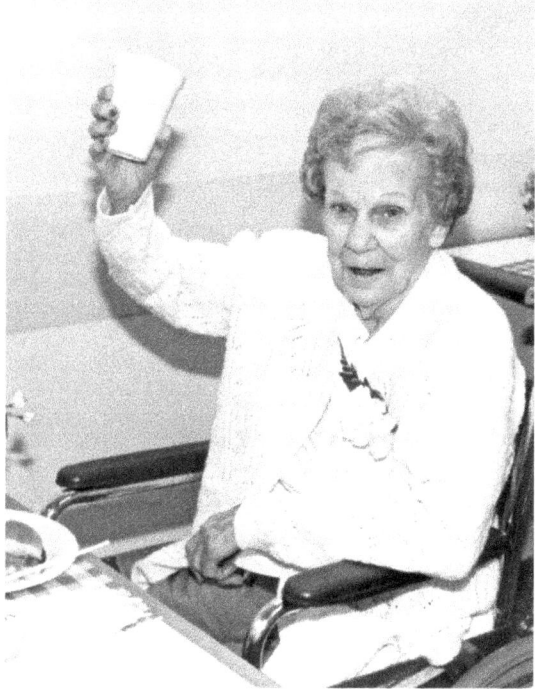

Right: Frances Weber, nursing home resident, toasts the staff at the anniversary picnic in 1994. *Courtesy of Valley Care Association.*

Opposite: Poster for Sewickley Antique Car Show, 1994. *Courtesy of Valley Care Association.*

VCA's programs. Gloria Berry, marketing consultant, directed publicity and advertising. "We had TV reporters riding around in antique cars," she said.

After the show, drivers headed out in a parade of cars to the nursing home to join a party reuniting old and new employees and trustees. Residents enjoyed an outdoor anniversary picnic the next day.

EXPANSION AND IMPROVEMENTS

Priorities outlined in the 1995 five-year plan were to add private rooms to the nursing home, more space for operations and privacy, more bathing facilities, and more space at the nursing stations and administrative areas.

Resulting changes included:

- Eight new beds for occupancy
- New furniture for the living room
- Electric beds for all rooms
- New furniture for the Staunton Wing

- A therapy space and a private dining room for residents and their families
- New lifting equipment for non-ambulatory residents to reduce the risk of back and neck injuries to the staff
- A snack cart to visit residential areas
- Thirty-six more parking spaces and a repaved sidewalk and driveway

DONATING BEDS TO NICARAGUA

When Valley Care replaced its old "crank" beds with new electric beds in 1994, residents were able to adjust their beds themselves, sit up in bed and perhaps get a drink of water. Nurses were relieved from the physical stress of having to crank beds up and down.

VCA trustee Dr. Robert Doebler told Dr. Olu Sangodeyi, his colleague at SVH, about the new beds. Sangodeyi suggested donating the 128 old beds to needy hospitals in Nicaragua. Doebler contacted Global Links, a Pittsburgh non-profit that delivered medical materials to aid developing countries. Global Links coordinated the delivery and found a donation of mattresses to go with the beds.

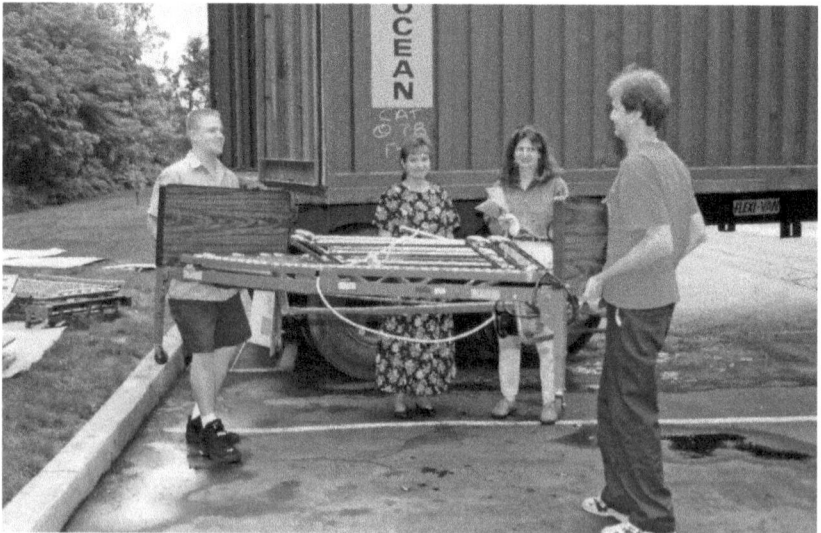

Valley Care Nursing Home employees Dave Baker and Dave Putt prepare beds for donation, helped by Lynn Harvey, director of housekeeping, and Kathleen Hower, executive director of Global Links. *Courtesy of Valley Care Association.*

BOARD MEMBER PROFILE: J. ROBERT FERGUSON JR.

J. Robert Ferguson Jr. was active on the VCA board from 1980 until 1996 and served as president from 1981 until 1987.

"One of the most impressive things about Robert Ferguson's service was the amount of time he put in," said Ellen Wright, VCA board secretary.

Ferguson joined the VCA board just prior to his retirement from U.S. Steel, where he was senior vice president and assistant to the president. "Valley Care became my retirement occupation," he said in 1987.

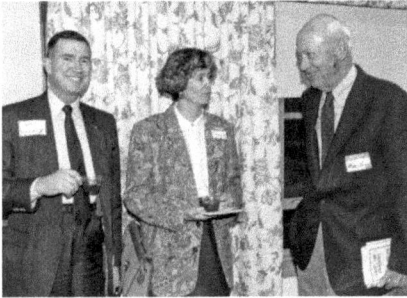

At the 1993 VCA annual meeting, board members Karl Ludwig and Dr. Lonnie Marshall exchange ideas with VCA president Robert Ferguson. *Courtesy of Valley Care Association.*

Ferguson was also a trustee at Sewickley Valley Hospital, chairman of the Sewickley Parking Authority and a director for ACTION Housing Incorporated (a nonprofit to promote housing for low- and middle-income families).

He and his wife, Dorothy, were chosen as *Sewickley Herald* Citizens of the Year in 1987. Robert Ferguson died on January 13, 1996, at age eighty.

5

Connecting with the Community, 1984–98

To give aid and comfort to the residents, a tremendous challenge. If you have ever had a loved one in a nursing home, you will appreciate the difference we can make.
—Valley Care Auxiliary mission statement

Neighbors Helping Neighbors

On a local level, Valley Care Association provided care for seniors and created a community. Many local people contributed by supporting VCA fundraisers, antique shows and other events.

Schoolchildren came in groups to sing and perform music for the elderly residents. Some of the other community groups that entertained residents or brightened the décor for the holidays included local clubs, churches, garden groups and animal humane societies.

VCA was also an active member in state and regional organizations that provided solutions for seniors. This involvement ensured that VCA remained abreast of the most current elder-care practices.

But primarily, for many area residents, Valley Care Nursing Home was where Mom, Grandma or Grandpa lived—in easy visiting distance for their children and grandchildren. Their closeness to home kept familial ties and traditions strong.

THE VALLEY CARE AUXILIARY

In May 1984, two months after the nursing home opened, Betty March was part of a group of women asked to form a VCA Auxiliary. March's vision and enthusiasm, coupled with many hours of hard work, was largely responsible for the rapid development of the organization.

In a September 1984 letter to current and prospective members, Dale Ryan, the first VCA Auxiliary president, set the organization's purpose: "to give aid and comfort to the residents, a tremendous challenge. If you have ever had a loved one in a nursing home, you will appreciate the difference we can make."

The first VCA Auxiliary meeting was held at the nursing home on September 28, 1984, to plan the activities of the year. Karen Davis, Valley Care Nursing Home activities director, gave a talk about "The Problems of the Aging." During the next twenty years, auxiliary members regularly heard from a number of experts on issues affecting older adults.

The auxiliary was officially established on October 30, 1984, with 150 members and 100 volunteers. It would grow to 200 members by 1986.

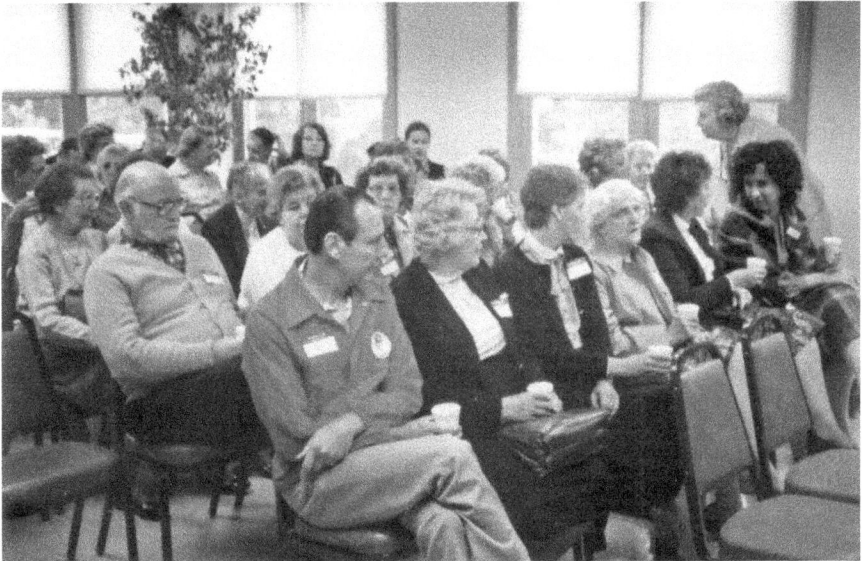

The first meeting of the Valley Care Auxiliary was held on September 28, 1984. *Courtesy of Valley Care Association.*

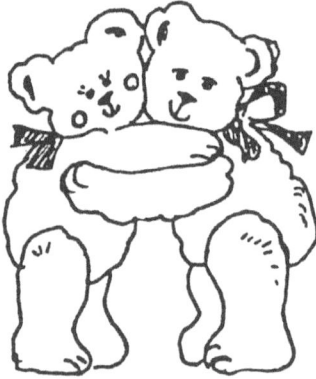

VALLEY CARE

AUXILIARY

Left: Valley Care Auxiliary logo was a symbol of friendship and caring, appearing on invitations and flyers. *Courtesy of Valley Care Association.*

Below: The Valley Care Auxiliary bake sale in 1997 was supported by Sewickley area residents Gordon and Dottie Price, Peggy Robinette and Hanna Wedeen. *Courtesy of Valley Care Association.*

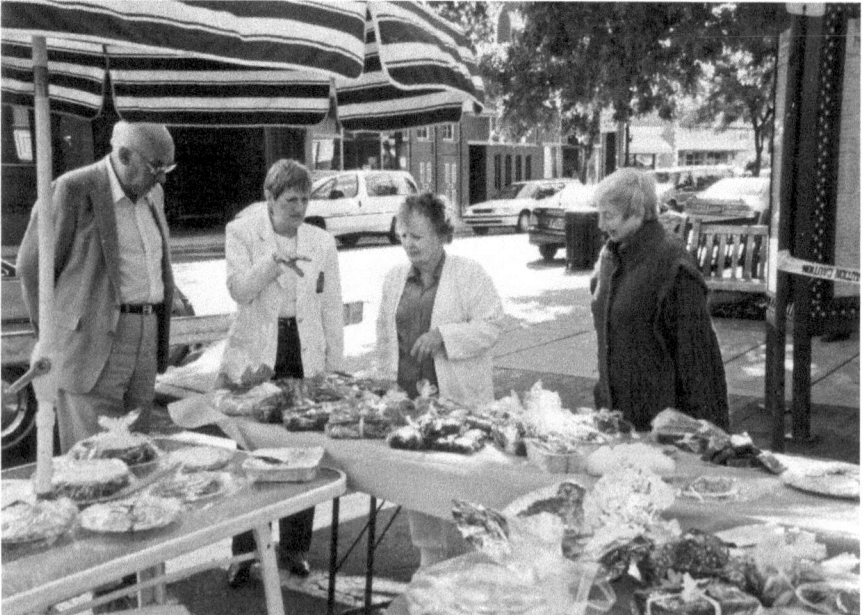

The officers in 1984–85 were:

Dale Ryan, president
Betty March, vice president*
Charlotte Benz and Nancy Burtch, treasurers
Anne Stouffer, corresponding secretary
Florence Neely, recording secretary
Barbara Smith, director of volunteers
Nellie Burrows, historian
Mrs. Stanley Briller, publicity chair

*Bobbie Booth became vice president when March died at age sixty-five on January 13, 1985.

Auxiliary members did more than volunteer their time. They organized major fundraising efforts to support the needs of the nursing home and the adult day care center. Auxiliary meetings often included lunch, an afternoon of cards, a fashion show or a speaker. These activities added a social aspect to the organization, building friendships and keeping members involved.

"I started with the auxiliary before the nursing home was built," said Gwen Ogle, auxiliary president in 1991. "We did fundraisers, the Care Fair at Christmas, and the antique show in September. We raffled off antique furniture. Sewickley had a lot of people who wanted [the furniture]—and a lot of people who wanted to get rid of it."

FUNDRAISERS SUPPORT ACTIVITIES AND CARE

The auxiliary's first project was the Care Fair, where it sold homemade crafts and unique boutique items made by residents and auxiliary members. It became an annual event held at the nursing home for one week at the beginning of the holiday season. The fair raised more than $30,000 over five years.

Starting in 1985, the auxiliary held an Appreciation Tea for nursing home volunteers during National Volunteer Week in April. It honored those who gave more than one hundred hours of service. This tradition continued for many years.

Mrs. Ray Albrecht and Mrs. Harton Semple led the auxiliary's effort to solicit advertising and print a Sewickley area telephone book. Sales of the phone book, along with advertising revenue, raised $13,159 for the

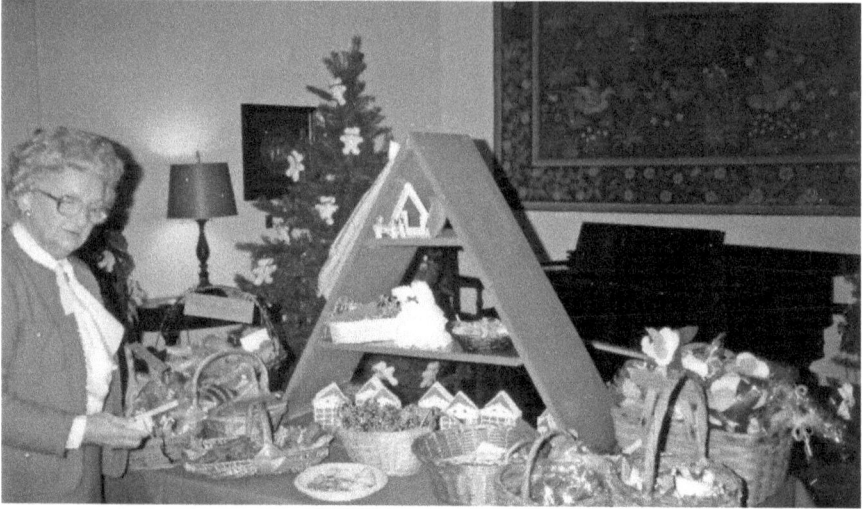

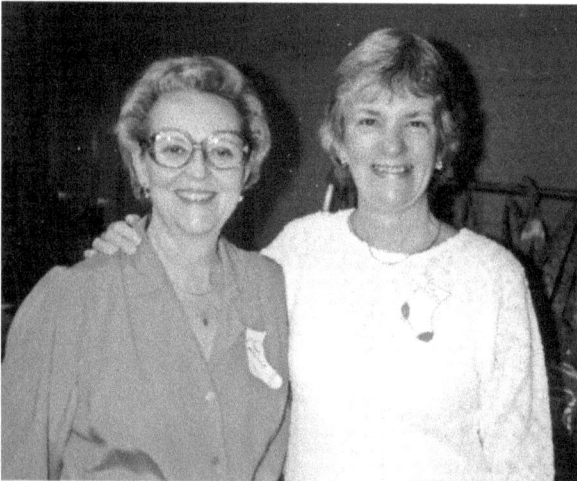

Above: Crafts for sale at the auxiliary's Care Fair were on display in the nursing home. *Courtesy of Valley Care Association.*

Left: VCA trustee Jean McClester (*left*) thanks Sue Harvey, co-chair of auxiliary's 1986 Care Fair for doing a great job. *Courtesy of Valley Care Association.*

auxiliary in 1989. A second volume was published in September 1993 and sold for $8 per copy.

The auxiliary donated $300 in 1989 to support an excursion for twenty-four residents who went "cruising down the river" in Pittsburgh on a Gateway Clipper ship. "The residents were excited, alert, and truly enjoyed themselves," said Ann Beck, activities director, in her thank you letter. "Your commitment to add so many 'extras' for our residents makes a big difference in their lives."

Another memorable fundraising event was the auxiliary's Great Sewickley Antique Fair and Collectible Flea Fair. The first one was held on the grounds

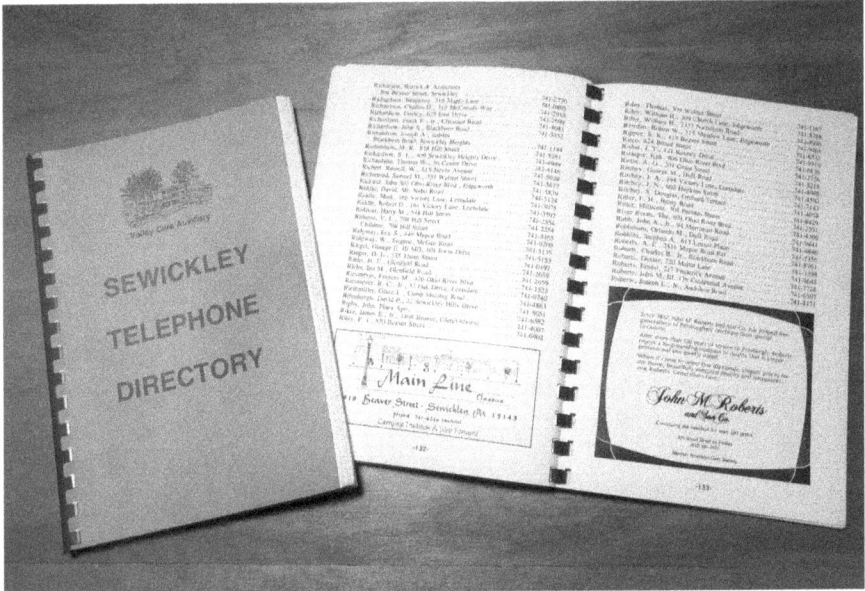

Above: The auxiliary held many fundraisers, including production and sale of the Sewickley phonebook. *Courtesy of Valley Care Association.*

Left: This flyer advertised the 1986 Antique Fair put on by the auxiliary. *Courtesy of Valley Care Association.*

THE GREAT SEWICKLEY
ANTIQUES FLEA FAIR

DEER RUN ROAD, SEWICKLEY PA.
AUGUST 30, 1986
9 AM — 4 PM

ADMISSION — $1.00

OVER 50 QUALITY DEALERS
SEWICKLEY AMATUER AREA
APPRAISAL BOOTH
INTERESTING FOOD

(412) 741 - 2281

From Sewickley - East on Beaver Street,
Lf. on Glen Mitchell Rd., Rt. on Merriman Rd.
Interstate 79 South - Sewickley Exit (No. 19)
Interstate 79 North - Glenfield Exit (No. 19)
Route 65 to Interstate 79 Exit

Follow Signs To Fair

Proceeds Benefit
Valley Care Nursing Home & Day Care Center

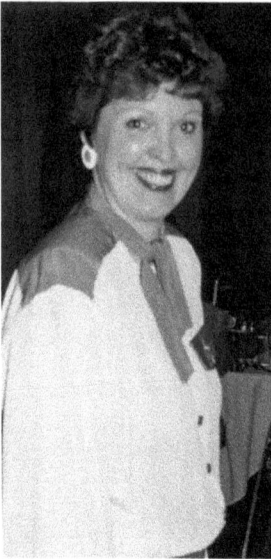

Ann Beck was director of volunteer and recreational services for the nursing home. *Courtesy of Valley Care Association.*

of the nursing home on August 30, 1986. For one-dollar admission, twenty-five hundred people browsed through wares from sixty dealers from three states. The flea market was set aside for amateurs who were told to "clean out their attics" and bring items to sell. Minta Roberts Bauer was chairman of the first fair.

The next year, the antique fair expanded considerably, with one hundred dealers from the tri-state area. More than four thousand people attended the event in Sewickley Heights Park on September 5, 1987. Items for sale included wicker, country furniture, linens, baskets, glass, tins and toys.

The 1988 Great Sewickley Antique Fair at Sewickley Heights Park charged $3 for admission. Even though a rainy forecast decreased attendance by about one-third, the event raised $6,000. Antique fairs continued for three more years.

In 1994, efforts focused on the antique car show in Sewickley Village. This event also became an annual fundraiser, with donated cars raffled off to raise additional funds.

In 1998, the auxiliary shifted gears and held a holiday house tour with the Sewickley Garden Council on November 28, at Tanna Flomer's house on Broad Street, Sewickley. Local interior decorators made donations to decorate rooms and sold the decorations at the end of the day. The auxiliary raised $3,200.

NEW FURNISHINGS ADD TO QUALITY OF CARE

The auxiliary purchased items that made life more pleasant and care easier for clients of the VCA Adult Day Care Center and residents of the nursing home. Some of these were "extras" that the facilities could not afford within their own budgets.

Items purchased in the first few years for the nursing home included furniture, refrigerators, typewriters, sewing machines, books, magazine and newspaper subscriptions and Christmas decorations. The Adult Day Care

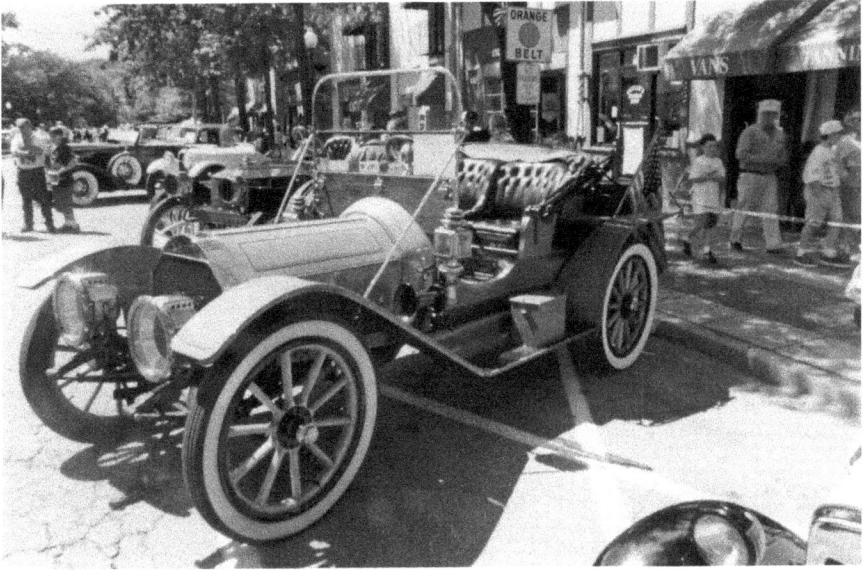

The antique car show was held on Broad Street in Sewickley in 1997. *Courtesy of Valley Care Association.*

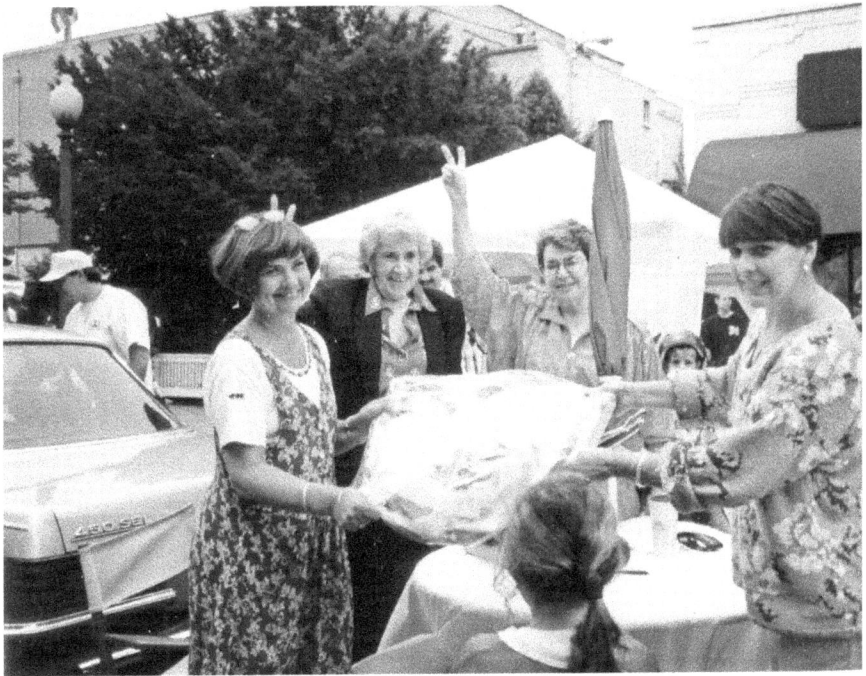

Valley Care Auxiliary members Paula Doebler, Pat Carton, Dorothy Urda and Pam Wright attend the Sewickley Harvest Festival in 1995. *Courtesy of Valley Care Association.*

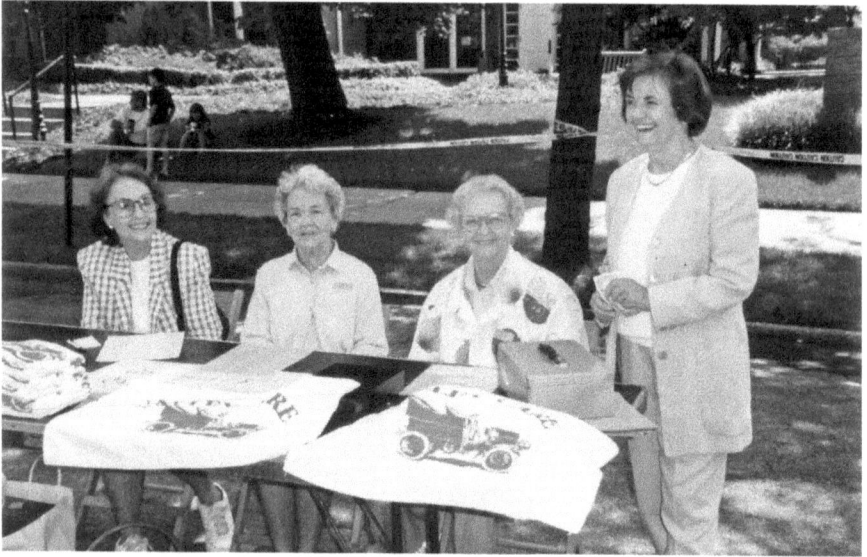

Valley Care Auxiliary members Gloria Berry, Virginia "Deedo" Ramsburg, Jean McClester and Marion Hayes staff the VCA table at the antique car show in 1997. *Courtesy of Valley Care Association.*

Center received outdoor and indoor furniture and a grill. Over the years, the auxiliary continued to donate furnishings and equipment to enhance activities, safety and comfort, including electronics, a Wander Guard personal security system, visits from a music therapist, a CPR instruction mannequin and a handicap-accessible swing.

One of the more substantial donations was $3,500 toward installing electric doors at the nursing home. The auxiliary also paid for the use of a swimming pool at the Verland Community Home, close by in Ohio Township, Pennsylvania, so nursing home residents could have swim therapy.

Subsequent donations to the Adult Day Care Center paid for re-covering furniture; a freezer, a microwave, small appliances and cooking equipment; decorations, games and prizes; a television and video cassette tapes; an intercom system; and air conditioning.

VOLUNTEERS GIVE PERSONAL ATTENTION

The volunteers at Valley Care Nursing Home offered a smile and a helping hand, lifting spirits to enhance the overall quality of life. They helped with recreation programs and made sure there were flowers on the tables. They assisted with personal care, filled water pitchers, delivered meals and pushed wheelchairs. Equally important, they read and listened to residents, making them feel that their lives still mattered. Volunteer service was coordinated and recognized by the Valley Care Auxiliary.

Volunteers who were honored during National Volunteer Week included:

- Margaret Grubbs, the auxiliary's first volunteer, who served 200 hours and specialized in visiting patients
- Mary Grazoli, age eighty, who volunteered for 200 hours mending sheets and bed pads from her home
- Evelyn McCall, the top volunteer in 1986, with 483 hours. She worked two days a week at the nursing home, eventually logging 2,380 hours of service. The McCall Award for outstanding service by a VCA volunteer was created in her honor.

Volunteers who received the McCall Award included:

- 1990: James Sims, Sewickley
- 1991: Margaret Grubbs, Aleppo Township
- 1992: Charles Bashaar, Franklin Park and Dale Umbel, Sewickley (honored for their woodworking classes)
- 1993: Nellie and Bill Burrows, Moon Township, with 3,681 hours
- 1994: Kay and Joe Bikowski, Leet Township, with 2,319 volunteer hours

---

VOLUNTEER PROFILE: HILDA SCHUSSLER

"Hilda Schussler is a special volunteer, as a resident of Valley Care Nursing Home in 1987 with nary a fault. Mrs. Schussler lends her creative talents to quilt making and her sewing ability to mending other residents' garments. A stich here, a hem there, loving thoughtfulness everywhere. Hilda was a resident of Osborne. What she is doing at her new home is just a continuation of what she did for many years for friends and neighbors."*

—Valley Care Newsletter

---

* *Valley Care Association Newsletter*, 1987.

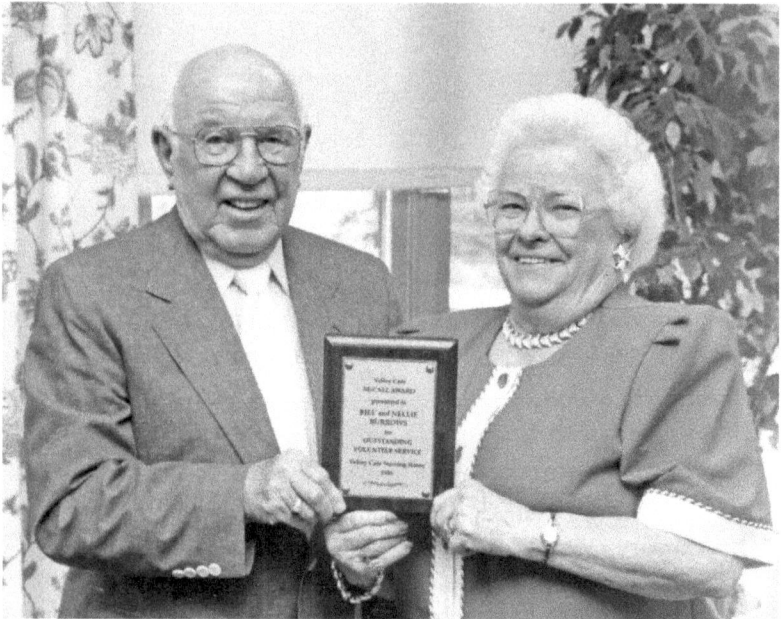

Volunteers Bill and Nellie Burrows were recognized in 1993. *Courtesy of Valley Care Association.*

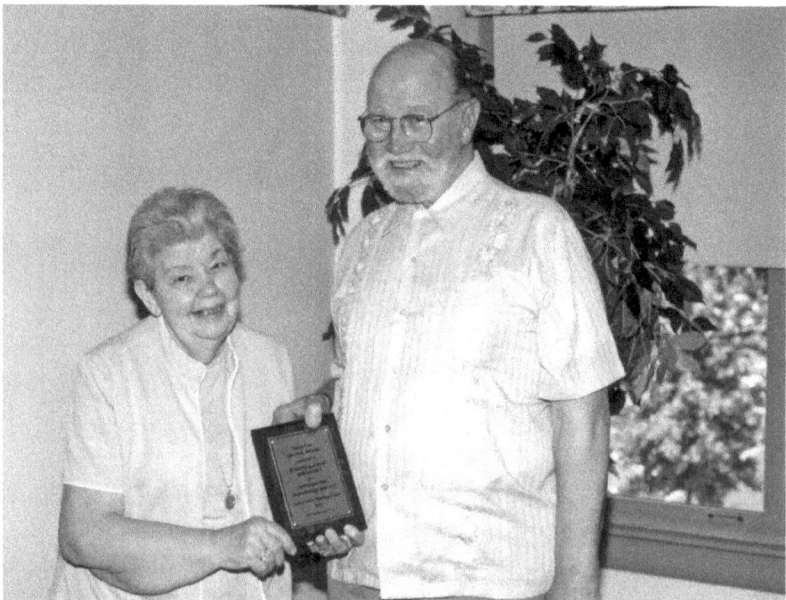

Kay and Joe Bikowski, Leet Township, were honored in 1994 for contributing 2,319 volunteer hours. *Courtesy of Valley Care Association.*

JOINING WITH OTHER COMMUNITY ORGANIZATIONS

Collaborations with other community groups often led to mutually beneficial alliances. One of the priorities of the 1994–95 five-year plan was to "encourage possible joint ventures to add community-based services complementary to Valley Care's mission."

In March 1993, VCA agreed to participate in a strategic long-term study initiated by Sewickley Valley Senior Citizens Services. The objective was to ensure that aging seniors in the Sewickley Valley could preserve their lifestyles. The board planned to analyze patterns of referrals from Sewickley Valley Hospital to Valley Care Nursing Home and donated $4,250 to the project.

In April 1995, the borough of Sewickley was selected by the Allegheny County Area Agency on Aging to try to develop an ElderCare Coalition of agencies, with possible ties to an SVH committee reviewing the needs of the elderly. VCA board members believed that supporting the ElderCare Coalition and interagency programs was an important priority.

ElderCare's vision was of a community committed to accessible, affordable and quality health care and opportunities for health improvement through prevention and education, with each agency having a role in making the vision a reality. The coalition reviewed gaps in existing services and implemented new programs and services to address those needs. The goal was to create awareness of new and existing services to support a healthier community through videos, brochures, a hot line, a community wellness kickoff day and community health education.

In 1996, the VCA board agreed to donate $4,500 to support the services of the ElderCare Coalition. A safety program held in May 1996 stressed in-home safety, with hundreds of area residents attending.

CONTRIBUTING TO THE CARING PROFESSION

VCA directors and administrators participated in professional organizations devoted to the improvement of elder care. They gave presentations, served as officers and spoke at conferences for groups, including:

- Quality Assurance Professionals of Western Pennsylvania
- Pennsylvania Adult Day Care Association
- Hospital Council of Pennsylvania

- Western Chapter of the Pennsylvania Association of Non-Profit Homes for the Aging
- Health and Welfare Committee of the Pennsylvania Senate and House
- Coraopolis-Sewickley chapter of American Association of University Women
- Robert Morris College (as part-time faculty)

One 1987 presentation featured Valley Care Nursing Home's Staunton Wing for Alzheimer's residents. Such invitations from state organizations recognized that the nursing home stood out in the field with something special to offer.

6

Changing Strategies for Changing Times, 1990–99

Does the sale meet our mission to serve the Sewickley Community? We are not currently meeting community needs because we don't have the money to build assisted living or additional adult day services. With the sale we will have money to adapt to changes in the community and meet their needs.
—James Alexander, VCA board president

In the 1990s, the Valley Care Association (VCA) faced ongoing financial challenges with reimbursement and the costs involved in keeping up its high level of care. The nursing home needed additional equipment, new technology and more services for a population that was increasingly older, more mentally confused and more physically fragile.

In 1992, board president James Alexander reported on the rollercoaster of operating a nursing home, which meant dealing with stringent Medicare regulations; rising health care costs in the United States; the uncertain future of reimbursement for Medicaid, Blue Cross and other insurers; and increased competition from other nursing homes. "The trend in hospitalization and nursing home care is toward greater consolidation of services, at lower costs," Alexander said in the 1992 annual report.

"It was hard to be a stand-alone facility with 120 beds," said Mary Mathews, director of social services and admissions for the nursing home. "We needed a continuum of care to feed people into the nursing home, and to provide all the services people want as they move from independent living to assisted living to nursing care."

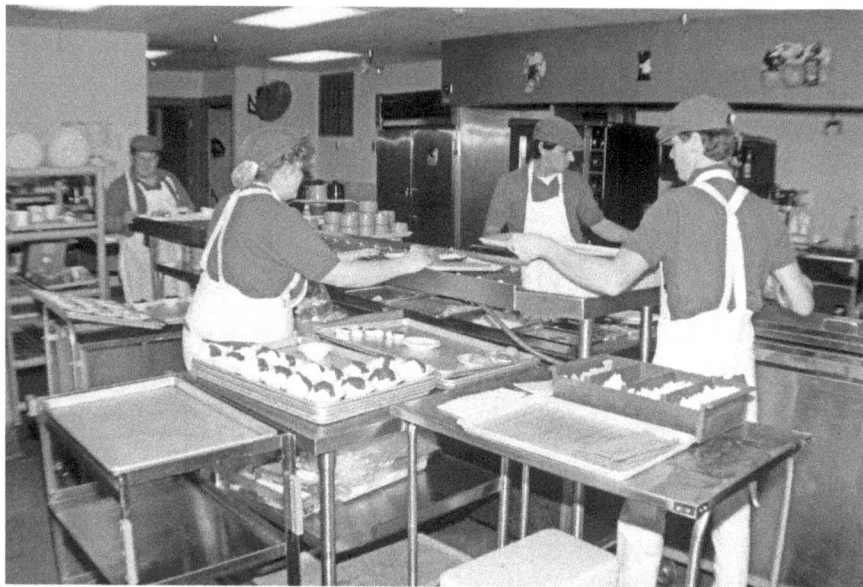

Above: Healthy, delicious meals were the goal of the dining department staff at the nursing home in 1992. *Courtesy of Ray Geffel.*

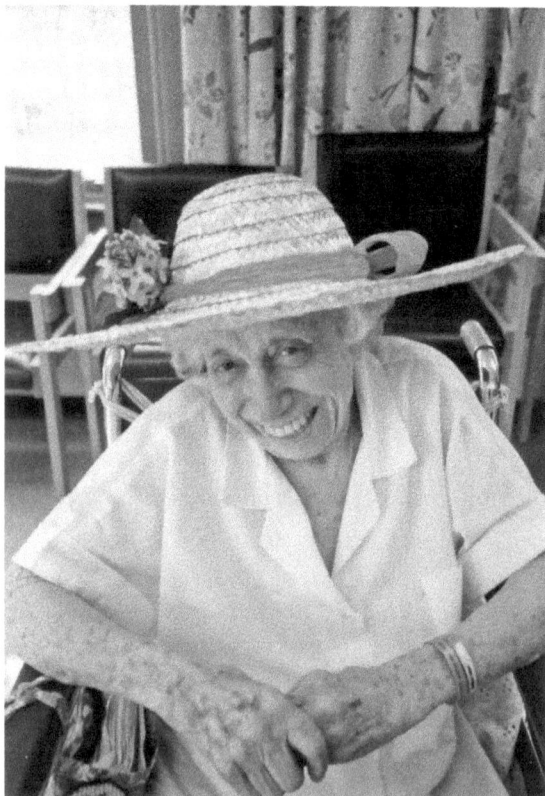

Left: Valley Care Nursing Home resident Anna Parry shows off her new straw hat in 1992. *Courtesy of Valley Care Association.*

At the 1994 annual meeting, Richard Lamden, president of the Jewish Association on Aging, presented a program called "Innovations in Long-Term Care." His talk touched on issues that would affect the future of Valley Care Nursing Home:

- The industry will be revolutionized by two trends: changes in technology and changes in the reimbursement system.
- Services will be provided in less-acute care settings—in long-term care facilities and in the growing industry of home-based services.
- Free-standing nursing homes will be a thing of the past as they become part of systems offering subacute, assisted living and specialty Alzheimer's care.

After a strategic planning session in January 1995, the board agreed to adopt a new long-range plan to:

- Maintain a primary commitment to improve the nursing home facilities, add more private rooms and increase space for operations and privacy
- Start to explore new services through task forces, starting with a senior resource referral service
- Encourage possible joint ventures to add community-based services complementary to VCA's mission
- Test fundraising potential for an assisted-living facility and new services

By July 1995, after reviewing the need for information and referral services, or a telephone reassurance program, board members agreed that other agencies, such as Contact Pittsburgh and the United Way, were already supplying these services.

EFFORTS TO CREATE A CONTINUUM OF CARE

While development of a nursing home was always a priority for VCA, the initial and ongoing mission was to offer a full range of care for older adults.

In October 1980, when the board voted to attempt the construction of a long-term care nursing home, it was described as "the first step in what it is hoped will later become a full retirement community, offering independent living and assisted living in addition to the skilled and intermediate services planned for the nursing home."

There was more than enough space for development on the land that surrounded the nursing home on Merriman Drive in Aleppo Township. Even during the first year of the nursing home's operation, VCA board members were working on plans for a retirement community for active seniors who wanted to live independently but without the burden of home maintenance. They would be able to remain close to Sewickley, surrounded by familiar faces and green landscapes. They would have private homes, along with recreational activities, fitness facilities, dining options and a variety of programs and entertainment.

An assisted-living facility would offer a different level of care than a nursing home, focusing on people who did not need skilled nursing care but did need help with daily tasks, such as dressing and bathing. It would allow them to continue living in their community with a new support system that would be less costly than a nursing home. The arrangement would include meals, housekeeping, laundry, transportation and personal assistance, as well as activities and socialization.

Gauging Interest in a Retirement Community

In August 1984, VCA mailed 378 questionnaires to determine the level of interest in a retirement community. Seventy-two people returned surveys, with thirty-three people indicating they would consider making a $1,000 deposit. The board considered this a positive response and began reviewing proposals from developers.

In January 1985, the board hired Retirement Centers Group (RCG) of Stamford, Connecticut, as developer of the retirement community. "We have assembled an outstanding team," said G. Whitney Snyder, vice president of VCA. "We look forward to providing an excellent environment for our friends and neighbors who are approaching retirement."[19]

VCA opened an office in Village Commons on Broad Street in Sewickley on March 1, 1985. The office established a presence in downtown Sewickley to market the retirement community and was open to "visits from local people who are potential retirement community residents to find out what amenities and services they want."[20]

PARTNERSHIP PROPOSALS

Over the span of twenty years, VCA considered eight proposals, including six serious attempts to connect with a developer or partner to create this continuum of care:

1985: Retirement Centers Group Incorporated, a retirement community with 160 to 180 apartments

1986: American Health Capital Development Company, as a joint project with Sewickley Valley Hospital

1988: PersonaCare, an assisted-living facility with 107 units on 5.5 acres

1990: Greystone Communication, a for-profit proposal not accepted by VCA

1995: Karrington Homes, an assisted-living facility with 60 units for up to 74 people

1996: Tandem Health Care, a for-profit proposal not accepted by VCA

1997: Valley Health System joint project

1999: Masonic Homes, which purchased and continues to operate the nursing home, along with a retirement community and an assisted-living facility

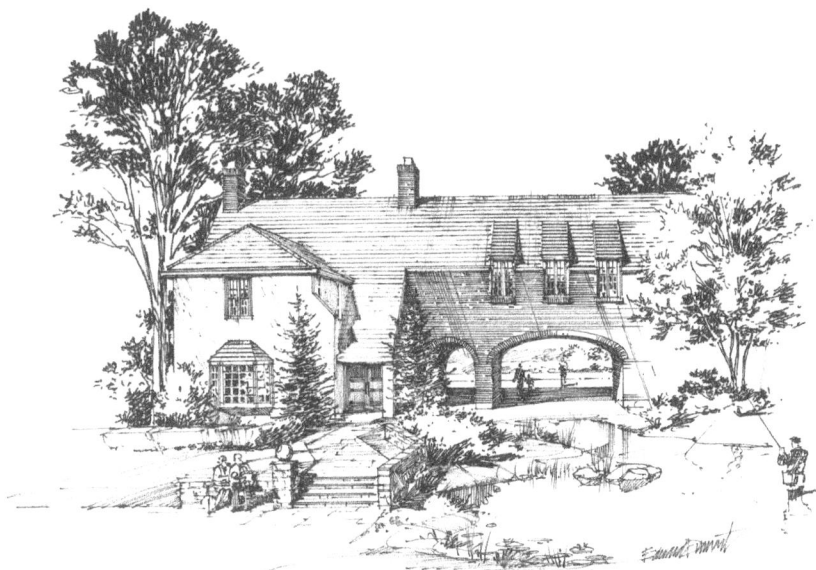

This concept for a VCA retirement community was designed by architects IKM SGE Incorporated. *Courtesy of Valley Care Association.*

In 1985, Betts Moore, director of development for VCA, conducted a pre-marketing survey for the proposed retirement community. "We want this community to be designed by those who are moving into it," she noted. "The housing needs to accommodate these individuals' present needs and lifestyles."[21]

RCG, however, had difficulty making a financial commitment to the project. In August 1985, two months before the project deadline, the board discussed RCG's inability to produce a viable project. The agreement was abandoned, but the goal remained.

A JOINT PROJECT WITH SEWICKLEY VALLEY HOSPITAL

The next attempt, in July 1986, was a joint project between VCA and SVH. Called the Elderly Housing Project, it was submitted by the American Health Capital (AHC) development company.

VCA signed an agreement with SVH in January 1987, to form a jointly owned not-for-profit organization to construct and operate a retirement community. The agreement authorized financing, land use and repayment of the loan from the proceeds.

The plan included:

- A mix of 150 independent-living units plus 30 personal care units
- SVH to be the owner of the development
- Valley Care to mortgage its forty acres and, hopefully, raise $400,000

It would take $800,000 to initiate marketing and six months to pre-sell units and arrange for zoning, sewage and road permits. By April 1987, SVH's finance committee decided it could not put its financing at risk. VCA considered other developers or continuing with the project as an independent venture but did not follow through with either option.

SHIFTING FROM RETIREMENT HOUSING TO ASSISTED LIVING

Based on these experiences, the VCA board shifted its expansion plans to creating an assisted-living/personal care facility that would give residents basic support services but not nursing care. Without the need to market a retirement community, VCA moved out of its expensive office in downtown Sewickley in August 1988. The board conducted business out of an office within the nursing home.

In January 1989, the board reviewed a proposal from PersonaCare of Baltimore to build a 110-room assisted-living facility on 5.5 acres of property that would be leased by Valley Care. The goal was to be open by fall 1991.

Board president James Alexander toured PersonaCare facilities in Chicago and Connecticut and was "impressed by the facilities themselves and the spirit of both residents and staff." PersonaCare staff surveyed the Aleppo Township property near the nursing home, conducted soil tests and worked on regulatory approvals and architectural planning.[22]

In October 1989, PersonaCare showed off a 3-D model of the facility, to be called "Sewickley Residence." By the next year, however, PersonaCare cut the number of units from 110 to 70, saying the market didn't seem favorable. In October 1990, PersonaCare backed out of the project, having been advised by its financial backers to fill the facilities it currently owned before starting any new projects.

DELAYED BUT NOT ABANDONED

Over the next few years, VCA remained committed to the assisted-living project that was "delayed but not abandoned."

In 1995, board members made a visit to Karrington Homes in Columbus, Ohio. Karrington's proposal was to build and operate a fifty-five- to sixty-unit assisted-living facility on VCA's property in Aleppo Township. VCA would contribute the land but not own the facility.

VCA's board resolved to retain Karrington and agreed to pay $10,000 to begin the first two phases of the contract, including a market study and pre-development planning, costing $30,000. The board agreed to file a preliminary application (at a cost of $6,000) with the Department of Housing and Urban Development (HUD), which would assume the risk. The board paid Karrington Architects $4,000 to design the building.

In January 1996, Karrington ended the project because it was no longer interested in building in "a rural location," according to the VCA board minutes. Karrington returned the $10,000 retainer.

WHERE DO WE GO FROM HERE?

The board held a special meeting on January 29, 1996, to discuss the future of an assisted-listing facility. Some of the questions debated were:

- Should it be a separate organization or a joint venture?
- Should VCA sell, lease or give the land to someone else to build it, with an agreement that referrals come to the nursing home?
- If it was a separate, self-supporting facility, was it still the board's responsibility?
- Did VCA's mission of caring for the aged fit this project?
- Could an assisted-living wing be added to the nursing home?

In discussing the risks, board members pointed out:

- There were too many uncertainties to justify a large facility.
- At $57 to $110 a day, it was too costly.
- The debt level would be excessive, and there was not enough money in the community to support it.
- The HUD process for approvals was cumbersome and would take years.
- The project would drain funds that the nursing home needed for renovation or would tap into the endowment funds.

Over the years, the board strived to stay true to the intentions of VCA's founding members. But how far did that responsibility extend over time as circumstances changed? The board also had a duty to consider the mission in the present context and to protect existing assets, services and clients from financial hardship.

In the end, the board agreed that although there was a great need for assisted living, as part of the continuum of care and to generate referrals to the nursing home, it was not financially feasible with seventy beds, as had been proposed previously, but perhaps would be as something smaller.

DISCUSSIONS WITH A HEALTH SYSTEM

On April 26, 1997, following two strategic planning sessions, the board resumed discussions about a merger or joint affiliation with Valley Health System (VHS)—the entity resulting from the merger of SVH and the Medical Center of Beaver. (This organization later became Heritage Valley Health System.)

Becoming a part of VHS would provide VCA with financial and managerial benefits, as well as the chance to share VHS's expertise in marketing, finance, management and information systems. In addition, an affiliation could result in an enriched system of health care providers and a large pool of potential donors.

Though VCA hoped to be tied into the new organization, VHS was occupied with making the hospitals' merger work and was slow to commit to giving VCA seats on the board. It could not define its intentions for long-term care and services for the elderly.

In August 1998, Tandem Health Care proposed an extensive, for-profit residential care campus with assisted- and independent-living alongside the Valley Care Nursing Home. The board minutes noted that VCA was not intended to be a for-profit entity.

"We have gone nowhere in four years, and our founding fathers wanted to develop the continuum," said Jane Tumpson, president of the VCA board.

It wasn't until September 1998, that a knowledgeable, capable and financially strong non-profit organization appeared on the scene. It brought a solution that would establish assisted living and a retirement community while continuing the nursing home—fulfilling the original vision of VCA.

EXTENDING THE RANGE OF SERVICES
WITH THE MASONS

The long trail of failed attempts was testament to the fact that the economic and geographic realities of the Sewickley Valley area did not favor a retirement community.

"We realized that we were too short of population. In a 20-mile radius around Sewickley, we had a high percentage of old people but not a high density," said former VCA board president Marvin Wedeen. "Three to five percent of people over 65 would need a retirement community, but that didn't get us enough people to be an economically viable unit. We had invited different private companies to come in and see if they would be interested in taking this over, and most of them saw the same thing we did. They backed away. They encouraged us, and then they kind of fell apart," he said.

"The Masons had a different perspective. They had a very extensive retirement community in Elizabethtown, [Pennsylvania] and they decided that they wanted to expand geographically. But the state had a limit on how many nursing homes they would allow. So the Masons were interested in buying our license, our nursing home, and our land to build a continuing care retirement community."

THE HIGH STANDARDS OF MASONIC HOMES

The Masonic Homes of the Grand Lodge of Pennsylvania started its Elizabethtown community in 1910. It was a community service organization that operated a not-for-profit continuing care retirement community and a children's home. In 1998, there was a three-year waiting list to buy into a Masonic Home retirement community.

Masonic Homes had the highest retirement community ranking in the nation by Standard & Poors, representing a deep commitment to maintaining high standards. It also had a long tradition of benevolent care, and residents were never asked to leave because they couldn't continue to pay the monthly fees.

Valley Care Masonic Center would be the fourth location, joining Elizabethtown; Masonic Eastern Star Home-West in Bellevue, Pennsylvania (eight miles from Sewickley); and Masonic Eastern Star Home-East, in Warminster, Pennsylvania (northwest of Philadelphia). When the Masonic Homes could not acquire Medicaid certification for additional beds at the Masonic Eastern Star Home-West, it looked for another way to provide services to people, regardless of their financial means.[23]

Joseph Murphy, executive director of Masonic Home of Elizabethtown, came to meet with VCA's board in September 1998. He said the Masons wanted to expand by buying a high-quality nursing home and chose this area as one that would attract people who wanted to be relatively close to a city.

They were aware that the Aleppo Township campus had been part of a larger vision by VCA to offer a continuing care retirement community. Masonic Homes shared this vision, making the transaction an ideal opportunity for both organizations.

The plan was to move forward by January 1999 and to build a sixty-unit assisted-living facility and independent-living housing by 2001. The Masons had a comfortable endowment and provided a lot of free care, Murphy told the board, "The purchase could be a cash deal. Proposals can be made for the protection of our mission and Valley Care's mission, with lots of room for negotiation."

The Masons planned to offer units to Masons, Eastern Star members and the local Sewickley community. "We made a deal with them that you didn't have to be a Mason to be a resident of the nursing home or community," said Wedeen.

"Does the sale meet our mission to serve the Sewickley community?" Alexander asked at the meeting. "We are not currently meeting community needs because we don't have the money to build assisted living or additional adult day services. With the sale we will have money to adapt to changes in the community and meet their needs."

Dan Peters, a VCA board member from 2003 until 2012, remembered the speculation surrounding the sale of the nursing home. "Why did we sell the nursing home? Some thought that what was originally built as a top-grade nursing home had fallen behind the industry standard in the quality of services it provided," he said. "VCA felt it could not grow laterally, so they turned it over to someone who could."

There was a consensus to proceed, as board members agreed that this "may be the last chance to generate funds to further our mission." According to the minutes, a letter of intent was signed on September 29, 1998.

INFORMING THE MEMBERSHIP AND COMMUNITY

VCA's board decided to reveal the Masons' proposal at the VCA annual meeting on October 26, 1998. In planning the invitation and agenda, the board minutes reported an agreement to "not use the words 'sale of the nursing home and property' as that gets people nervous. Instead, discuss the Masons' ability to build assisted living, their experience at Elizabethtown, and positive reputation."

Forty-two members attended the membership meeting. "Health care has been very different in the '90s than it was in the '80s," Tumpson said that day. "For the past two years, VCA has discussed the need to create a continuum of care and revised the vision and mission of the organization. We have increased our involvement in the community and discussed the future of the nursing home in this changing environment."

Tumpson told the audience that long-term care had become more complex, with residents needing more medical, psychological and emotional interventions than in the past. Valley Care Nursing Home's management was challenged by the need to admit residents twenty-four hours a day, seven days a week; deal with more regulatory standards and less reimbursement; and continue to provide high-quality care in a cost-effective manner.

"How do we survive in the future—stand alone or align with someone?" Tumpson asked the audience. "We have talked for 18 months with VHS to establish an affiliation or a merger, but those discussions stopped when VHS realigned their own board. We decided to look elsewhere and are talking to a nonprofit group that is interested in an affiliation, with a similar mission. These talks are continuing and we see this as a way to create an assisted-living or independent-living facility on the land, which was the original mission of our founders."

There was no negative feedback from staff or families.

The board met with the Masonic board on November 24 to discuss the purchase price, employee contracts, access to beds and other issues.

FINALIZING THE TRANSITION

The letter of intent drafted in December 1998, discussed the sale of the nursing home and land, property, plant and equipment. On March 17, 1999, the board accepted the final draft of the asset purchase agreement for $6 million for the nursing home and $1 million for the land.

VCA would have to pay off the nursing home debt. It would also need to cover about $100,000 for miscellaneous costs and legal fees, $77,000 for workers compensation and $100,000 for miscellaneous repairs or emergency costs. That left a possible net amount of $5.4 million.

VCA would keep the current accounts receivables and the existing endowment of $600,000. They also requested first right of refusal should the Masons wish to sell any of the land.

The first draft of the purchasing agreement was received on January 19, 1999. Minutes of the meeting that night stated that the agreement "looks good in general," and the goal was an April 30 or June 30 closing date.

The accounts receivable would cash out in six months. With current investments and other assets, the total net value was $8 million. The agreement and sale were also subject to the approval of the state's Department of Health, Department of Welfare and attorney general.

MEMBERSHIP AND AUXILIARY RESPONSE

At a special membership meeting on March 22, 1999, ninety-two members voted to approve a resolution to sell the Valley Care Nursing Home and surrounding property to the Masonic Homes of Elizabethtown, Pennsylvania. The board voted to approve the asset sale. Current employees would remain on staff, including nursing home executive director B.J. Franks.

The board clarified how VCA would operate following the sale:

- Its mission would be to facilitate services for the elderly in the community.
- The money from the sale would generate income to support programs for older adults in the Sewickley Valley region.
- Specific goals and objectives would be defined through a series of strategic planning meetings.
- Jane Tumpson would be appointed executive director of VCA.

With the pending sale of the nursing home, many Valley Care Auxiliary members felt they were without a purpose.

On March 2, 1999, auxiliary president Ruth Lessman wrote her members, saying, "The Association Board would like the Auxiliary to continue and to support the Adult Day Care Center in Ambridge. But this is our dilemma. In recent years, dues-paying membership stayed at close to 100, but very few were willing to work on fundraisers, and an average of 20 attend meetings." Soon after, the auxiliary asked for and received permission to dissolve. Its final membership meeting was on May 17, 1999.

On May 25, 1999, the VCA board of directors held its last meeting as the board of trustees of the nursing home. Formal closing on the sale of the nursing home and forty acres of adjacent land to Masonic Homes was set.

DEDICATING VALLEY CARE MASONIC CENTER

On June 1, 1999, at 5:00 p.m., following the formal closing of the sale, the Masons held a dedication ceremony, formally acquiring Valley Care Nursing Home and changing the name to Valley Care Masonic Center. VCA board members were invited to the unveiling, tours of the property with Masonic leadership and a social hour and dinner at the Allegheny Country Club.

"As we change the sign today, it is not a change of mission, but a forming of a partnership for progress serving the Sewickley Valley area," said James Ernette, grand master and chairman of the Committee on Masonic Homes.

"This is an emotional moment for the members of our community who were involved in the establishment of Valley Care in 1978," said Alexander. "This name—Valley Care Masonic Homes—unites the Masonic Homes and the Sewickley community in a way that not only is symbolic, but also reflects a relationship that will continue into the future."

The Masons' experience and existing facilities provided the expertise and economies of scale that would assure the ability of the nursing home to continue to serve the community and to realize the vision of VCA's founders for a true continuum of care.

DEVELOPING A RETIREMENT COMMUNITY

On September 24, 1999, the Committee on Masonic Homes approved the master plan for expanding the Valley Care Masonic Center into a continuing care retirement community, called the Masonic Village at Sewickley. The plan included a four-story, sixty-bed personal care facility connected to the Valley Care Masonic Center to be named the Star Points Building.

In addition to residents' rooms, Star Points featured a dining room, a great room, an assembly room, lounges, terraces, medical clinics, a beauty/barber shop, a pharmacy, a gift shop and a childcare center, at a total cost of approximately $14 million. Construction began in July 2000. On November 26, 2001, the first of forty residents moved from the Masonic Eastern Star Home-West into the new assisted-living building. The Masonic Homes closed and sold the Masonic Eastern Star Home-West.

The master plan also included a retirement community with 228 apartments, 35 villas, a clubhouse and a wellness center, at a cost of $63 million. The clubhouse contained a bank, general store, library, dining room, café, salon, lounge and computer resource center. Construction began in October 2001. In March 2003, residents started moving into the first apartments.

This style of retirement living appealed to Sewickley residents who no longer wished to maintain their homes and yards but still wanted to be close to their communities, churches, synagogues and former neighbors. As more of these neighbors moved to Masonic Village, they created a "second Sewickley" in Aleppo Township.

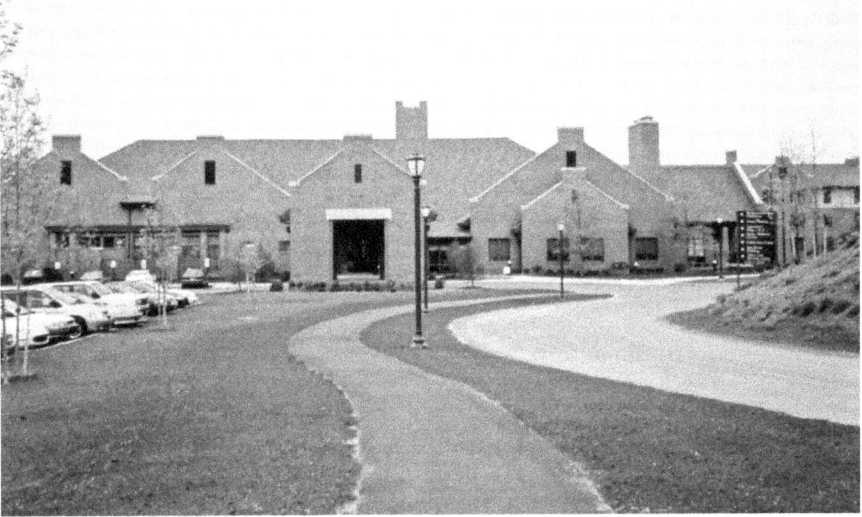

The clubhouse at Masonic Village housed dining and recreational facilities. *Courtesy of Valley Care Association.*

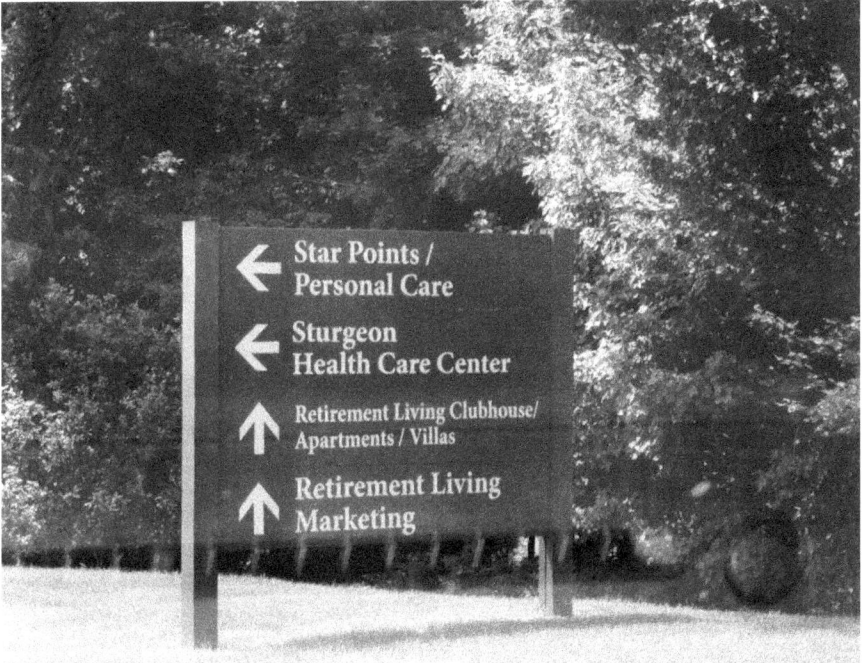

In 2014, Masonic Village renovated the nursing home and renamed it Sturgeon Health Care Center. *Courtesy of Valley Care Association.*

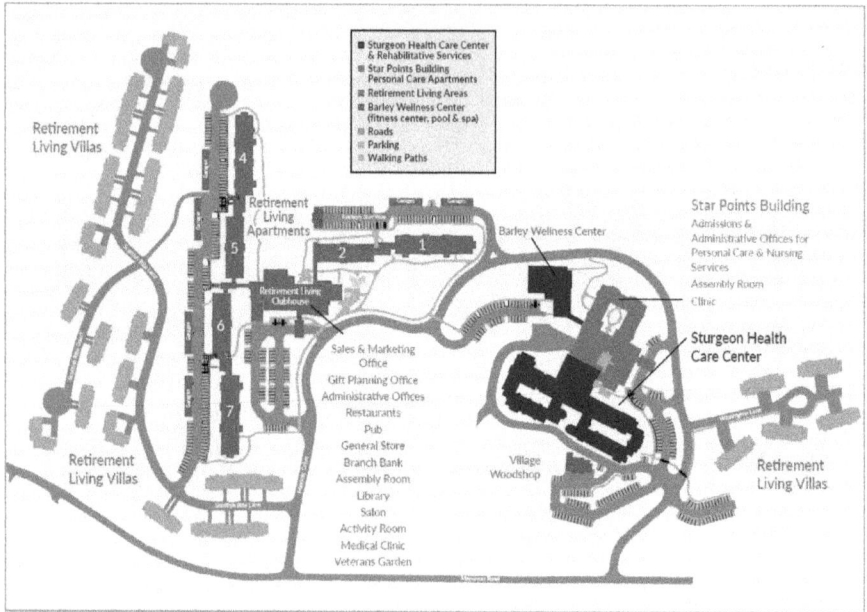

Masonic Village offered a wide range of housing options and facilities in 2018. *Courtesy of Valley Care Association.*

In 2002 and 2003, the Valley Care Masonic Center was renovated, and the Barley Wellness Center was built adjacent to the Star Points Building. The wellness center included a swimming pool, Jacuzzi and fitness facility. In 2006, eight additional villas were added.

In 2014, the Masons renovated the nursing home (now called the Sturgeon Health Care Center) and built a 66,000-square-foot addition. The building was laid out in eight sixteen-bed units called "neighborhoods," each with its own dining room, living room and parlor. There were eighty-eight private rooms and twenty private suites, with two dedicated memory-support neighborhoods and a transitional care unit for short-term rehabilitation. An assembly room was used for entertainment and special events and served as a chapel.

Over the years, Masonic Village acquired adjacent parcels of land. Construction began on ten new villas in 2018, with residents moving in during the second half of 2019.

Masonic Village at Sewickley meets the care needs of its residents throughout their lives, allowing them to move seamlessly from retirement living to the health care portion of the campus (if these services are ever needed). This continuum is known as a life care arrangement. When

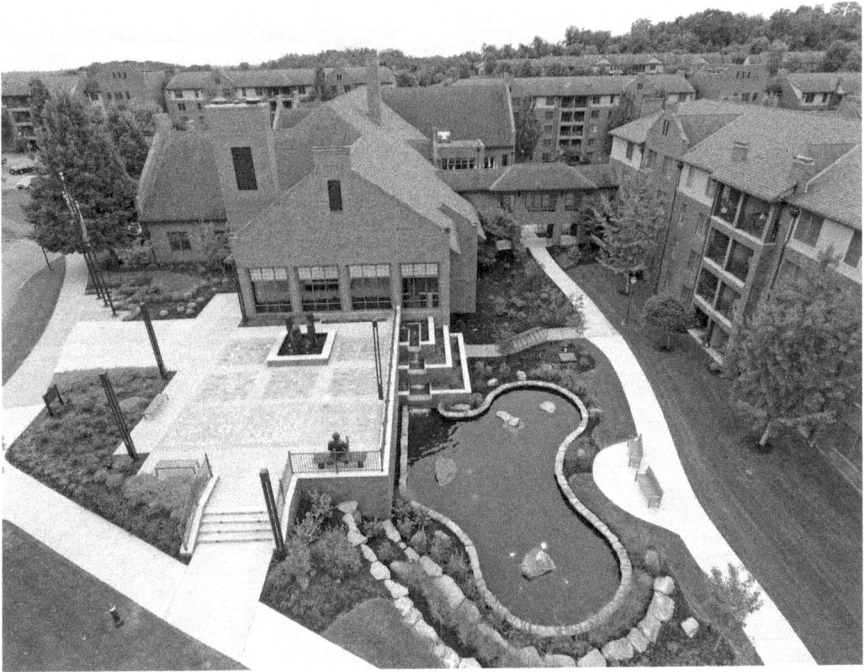

Masonic Veteran's Garden was designed to encourage activity and contemplation. *Courtesy of Richard Johnson, creative director for Masonic Villages.*

residents move to Masonic Village, they pay a one-time entrance fee and then a predictable monthly service fee that covers meals, maintenance, utilities, twenty-four-hour security and transportation to area stores and medical providers. This arrangement ensures the residents' monthly fee remains steady even if they require nursing or personal care services.

MASONIC VILLAGE CONTINUES TO THRIVE

In 2018, Masonic Village had approximately 500 residents. About 250 of them lived in one of six four-story apartment buildings, with 65 people living in forty-four villas. The remaining 185 were in the personal care or nursing home facilities. The minimum age to move in was fifty-five, but most residents were age seventy and older.[24] Masonic Village had four hundred employees, including part-time workers.

In 2018, sixty people lived in the Star Points Personal Care apartments and received meals, along with help with bathing, dressing and taking

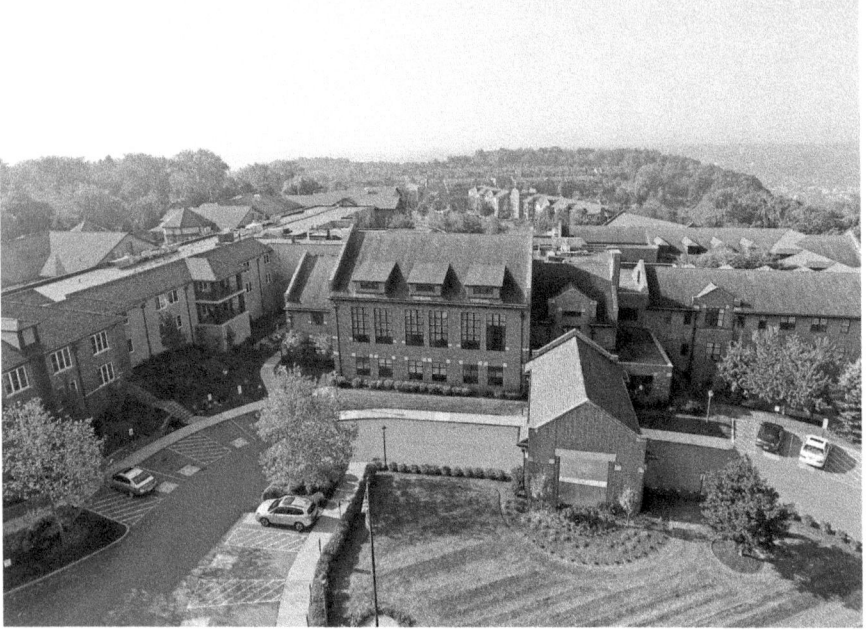

Masonic Village expanded its residential options to include apartments (pictured here) and villas for independent living. *Courtesy of Richard Johnson, creative director for Masonic Villages.*

medication. They often had physical limitations or dementia but did not need constant skilled nursing care.

Eric Gross, executive director of Masonic Village since 2009, joined the VCA board in 2011. His term as president was from 2017 until 2020. "The expansion of the VCA nursing home to what is now Masonic Village at Sewickley represents the realization of a long-range vision by VCA's founders to have a comprehensive retirement community available to older adults in this area," he said.

REINVENTING VALLEY CARE

Without the nursing home, VCA board members had to reconsider their goals and, eventually, adjust the structure of the organization.

The board held strategic planning sessions during the spring and summer of 1999 to develop a three- to five-year plan with goals and program objectives. Included was a review of the organization's values, governance, investment of assets, awarding of grants and bylaws.

In June 1999, VCA revised its mission statement to state its new objective:

Valley Care Association is a not-for-profit organization whose mission is to facilitate the provision of services to enhance the quality of life, primarily for senior citizens and older adults in our community.

In proceeding with its new mission, the board made a number of changes to restructure and move forward:

- Change the maximum number of trustees from twenty-nine to nineteen
- Strive for more geographical representation on committees
- Maintain an executive committee with a president, one vice president (instead of two) and a combined position of secretary/treasurer, including other directors as invited
- Create a grants committee that would be responsible for prospecting and reviewing proposals
- Take an active approach to seeking projects and activities to fund the Adult Day Services and Elizabeth G. Moore Scholarship Fund
- Take a passive approach with regard to investments
- Set investment parameters—no social issue constraints, just increase the principal with a risk tolerance of 10 to 11 percent

Over the next ten years, VCA would continue to enhance the quality of life for the elderly by expanding adult day care services, awarding grants, offering home repairs and joining with other community groups.

CHANGING STATUS AS A CHARITABLE ORGANIZATION

The total assets of VCA on June 30, 2000, were $9,405,410, including $8 million from the sale of the nursing home and additional funds from a generous bequest from the estate of Adie Ritchie. VCA members and community supporters redirected their donations from the Assisted Living Fund (which was no longer needed) to the VCA general endowment.

Two financial consulting firms, Salomon Smith Barney and Yanni Bilkey Asset Planning, were hired to help determine VCA's asset portfolio structure. Each was given $4 million to invest.

BOARD MEMBER PROFILE: JAMES ALEXANDER

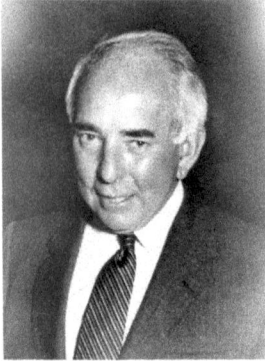

James Alexander was born in Toronto, Canada, in 1921. He worked at Shawinigan Chemicals in Quebec before joining Bayer in 1964 as president of Verona-Pharma Chemical in New Jersey. He served as senior executive vice president of Mobay in Pittsburgh and later as chairman of the board of Allegheny Plastics.

After retirement, he served on the VCA board from 1984 until 2004, becoming president in 1992 and again in 1999, when he shepherded the organization through the sale of the nursing home to Masonic Homes.

James Alexander. *Courtesy of Valley Care Association.*

He was married to Helen Alexander, and he also served as president of the Pittsburgh Blind Association. He died in 2009.

With the sale of the nursing home, the board reviewed VCA's legal status. In January 2000, it was a 509(a)(3)—defined as a supporting organization for the nursing home. Without the nursing home, it was reorganized as a 590(a)(2) charitable organization.

It could become a private foundation or remain as a public charity. To remain a public charity (beyond the eighteen months remaining in the current tax status at that time) it needed to pass the public support test, with an ongoing annual fundraising campaign that drew 10 percent of its annual income from the general public.

VCA retained its status as a public charity until November 2006, when it failed to meet the public support test because of its increase in investment income and decrease in public support. It would need to generate at least $300,000 annually in public contributions to retain that status. Instead, after much discussion, the board reorganized into two separate corporate entities:

- Valley Care Association became the operational body to make grants and work with programs that received funding, including the adult day services.

- The Valley Care Endowment (VCE)—legally a corporation— held and managed the investment portfolio and distributed funds for the benefit of the Valley Care Association.

In 2007, VCA transferred all assets to the Valley Care Endowment Corporation. VCE held its first board meeting on November 1, 2007.

VCE provided the funds to support VCA's grants to organizations serving the elderly. It also gave financial support to cover the ongoing deficit generated by the two Valley Care Adult Day Services centers.

7

Adult Day Care Services,
1982–Present

We empower individuals and caregivers of all ages to be active, safe, and healthy.
—VCA vision statement

While creating a nursing home was the Valley Care Association's (VCA) initial objective, a full continuum of care for older adults was always part of the plan. As early as 1978, the organization's goals included "offering the socialization and structure that seniors could be given through adult day services."[25]

As noted in chapter 2, health policy experts encouraged VCA to move ahead with its plans for adult day care programs for the elderly, even before the nursing home was built. Additional options would ensure that aging adults wouldn't be forced into nursing homes unnecessarily but could receive care at the level they needed.

VCA understood that it could help families struggling to keep aging loved ones at home. A day care center offered a number of benefits:

- A break for caregivers who needed to work and/or care for family members
- A degree of independence for seniors seeking to stay at home
- Activities and socialization for clients who attended the day care
- Support to families, if the caregiver was unavailable
- A less costly alternative to assisted living or a nursing home
- A transition or bridge to other long-term care
- On-site professional health care and other services

The Valley Care Adult Day Care Center (ADCC) raised the quality of life for the elderly participants, providing vital social interaction, maintaining health, and promoting independence. At the same time, their family members were able to continue working in or outside of the home.

"Socialization is so important," said Gwen Ogle, Valley Care Auxiliary president and VCA board member. "People need to be stimulated from when they are born until the time they die. Age has nothing to do with it. It is a necessary part of living."

According to Ogle, aging at home is not always the best option. If an older adult is alone, without visits from friends or family, they will deteriorate. Aides can help them be independent in their own homes, but adult day care provides more human contact, social connections and mental and physical activity.

"We know that a lack of socialization causes depression and chronic disease. They exhibit dementia that they don't have. People can die from a lack of stimulation, and that's one of the problems with the home health situation," Ogle said.

A Demand for Adult Day Care

In 1982, the outreach committee of the VCA board conducted a community survey on needs in the region for transportation, adult day services, information and referrals. In a few short months, the committee was looking into the purchase of a van and at the possibility of placing an ADCC in the Aleppo Township Municipal Building.

On January 20, 1983, the VCA board signed a lease with Aleppo Township. By February, renovations were underway. Continuing the spirit of community evident in all VCA activities, Sewickley Valley Hospital agreed to supply meals for the program. By March 30, Janice L. Pritchard was hired as director of the ADCC.

There were seven inquiries from interested clients even before the center officially opened on May 4, 1983, with four people attending. It was calculated that ten clients would be needed to break even. By the end of 1983, the site was operating within budgeted projections, with an average of thirteen clients. About 75 percent of ADCC clients were from the local service area.

A local newspaper reported that the center was "open four days a week from 9 a.m. to 3 p.m. The $15 [daily] fee covers two meals, crafts, and socialization. Reality therapy is conducted for confused clients, and

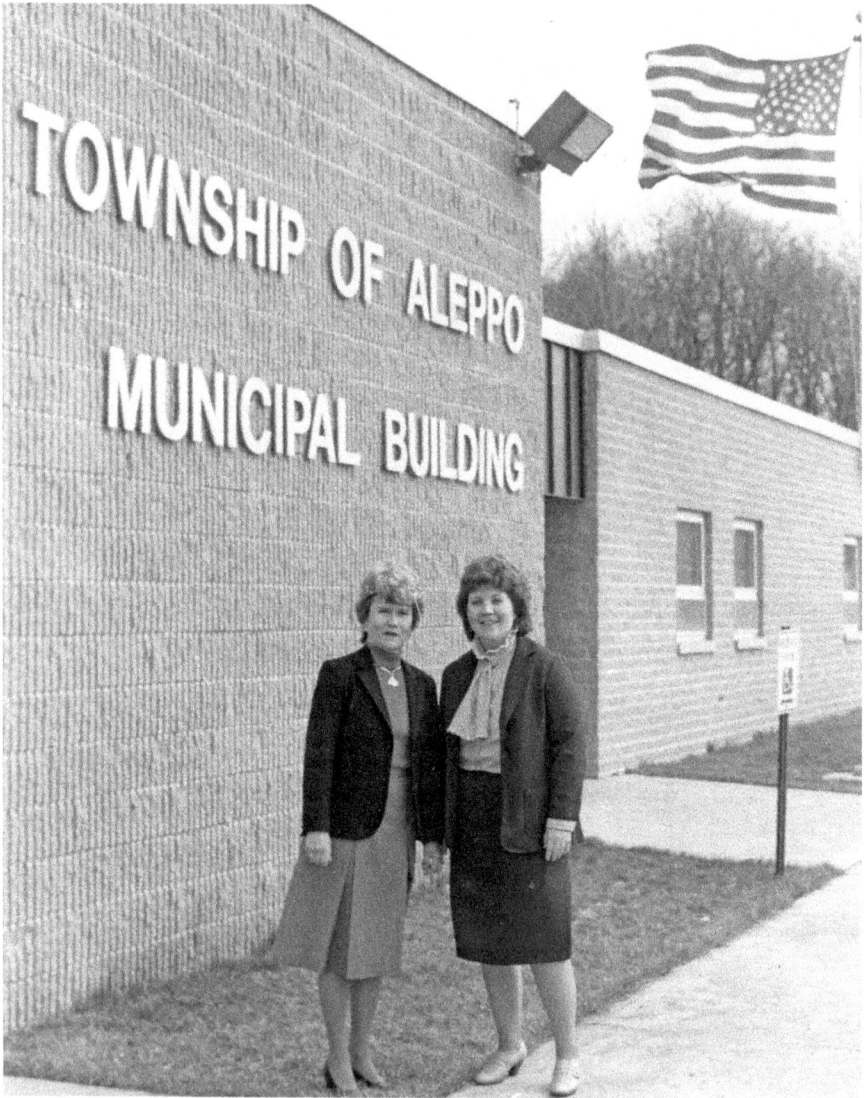

Board member Jane King (left) and Janice Pritchard, Adult Day Care Center director, pose outside the building that housed the center in 1983. *Courtesy of Valley Care Association.*

a registered nurse is on hand. There are facilities for 20 clients in the municipal building."[26]

"Most of the people I have now are parents being cared for by people who have already retired—a second generation of retired people," said Pritchard."[27]

PAYING FOR SERVICES

The daily fee would rise to between sixty-two and seventy dollars a day by 2007, a significant amount to be paid by the client, their adult children or a spouse—yet it still didn't cover all costs.

"No one disputes the value of adult day care services for the elderly, but today, without public funding or private insurance supporting it, it is not a viable financial option for most families," said VCE board member Dan Brooks, MD.

Over the years, the ADCC program experienced highs and lows with respect to attendance and income, affected by the weather, transportation issues and financial support from county organizations for the elderly. It never truly turned a profit but was by all accounts considered a success in fulfilling its mission.

"The ADCC revenue from private-pay or county-supported clients was never going to be enough to be self-sustaining," said VCA board member Dan Peters. "It was necessary to subsidize it indefinitely, especially as we had to have a first-class adult day care operation. Our services are high quality, providing mental and emotional stimulation and socialization. To do that, the subsidy [from VCA] is essential."

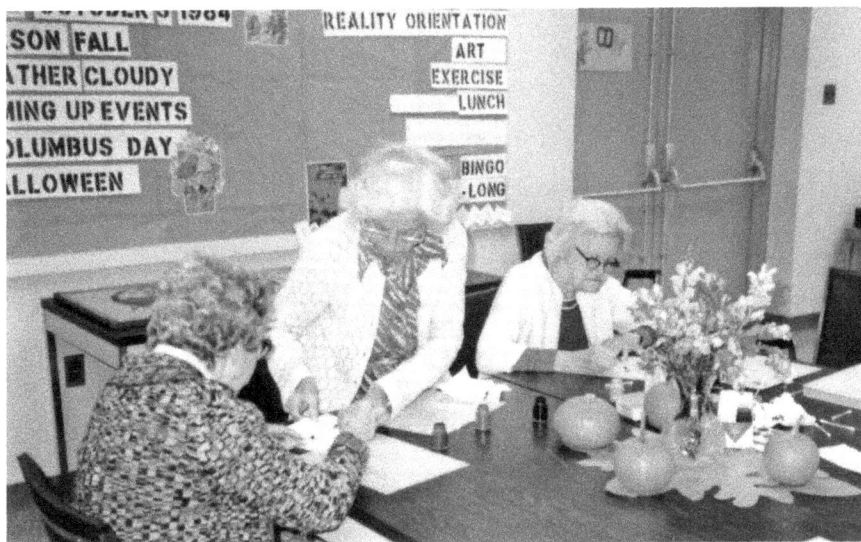

When clients made autumn crafts at the Aleppo Adult Day Care Center in 1984, they engaged their minds and their hands. *Courtesy of Valley Care Association.*

KEEPING CLIENTS ACTIVE AND HAPPY

The ADCC remained in the Aleppo Municipal Building from 1984 until 1989. Services were oriented around raising the quality of life for those who used the service, encouraging the participants to maintain their independence for as long as possible and to make the most of the years left in their lives.

Activities included local field trips and time spent outdoors, playing games and enjoying picnics. The seniors had a chance to continue hobbies, such as gardening in the center's small plot, which produced tomatoes, peppers and a variety of flowers. They had intergenerational programs with a local children's day care center, bringing seniors and children together, according to Kathi Miller, who was acting director of the ADCC from 1985 until 1989.

The center attracted community groups, including speakers from the Red Cross, American Cancer Society and Pittsburgh Blind Association. A dentist from Pitt Dental School brought each client a dental care kit. Even children from Youngworld Day Care Center in Franklin Park, Pennsylvania, presented a program of song and dance.

Holidays were celebrated with decorations, parties, costumes and special refreshments. In 1986, there were visits from the Easter Bunny and from

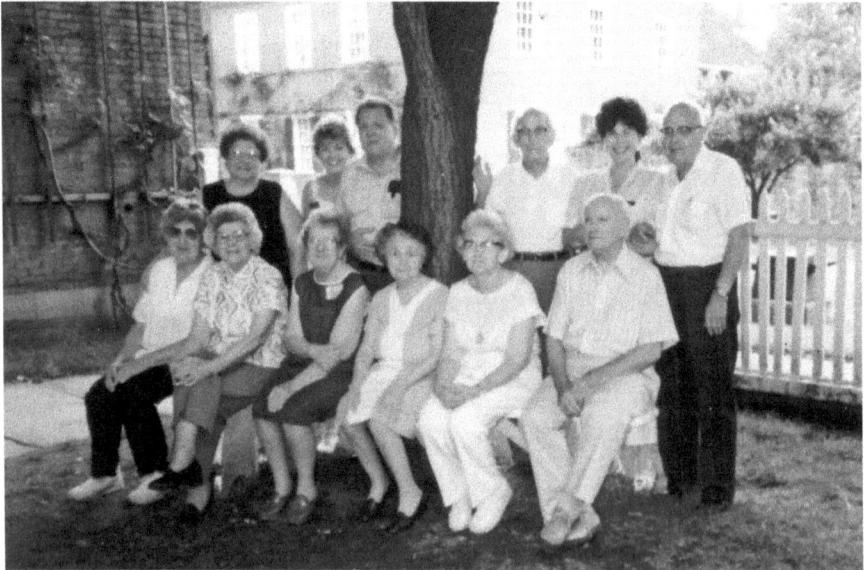

ADCC clients take a field trip to the Old Economy Village historical settlement in Ambridge in July 1987. *Courtesy of Valley Care Association.*

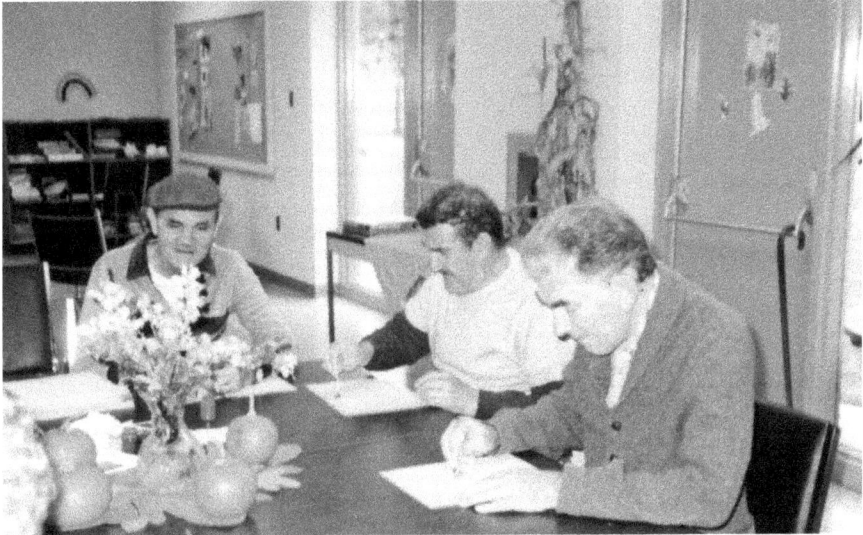

Seasonal arts and crafts helped clients connect socially at the Aleppo ADCC in 1984. *Courtesy of Valley Care Association.*

Halloween goblins from the Glen Montessori School, as well as a Christmas dinner with family members, complete with caroling.

In January 1984, with the number of client days on the rise, the VCA board signed an agreement with Crossgates (the management agent for the Valley Care Nursing Home) to supervise the ADCC for $100 a month until client days reached fifty per week. The agreement was short-lived, and the board decided to hire a new part-time director instead. Carol Benefield started on July 2, 1984, and stayed until August 31, 1985.

Over the 1984–85 fiscal year, the number of clients increased from thirteen to twenty, with the average weekly days used by each client growing from two to two and a half days. Many families claimed that they would like to use the service but couldn't drive their elderly relatives to the site.

VCA initially decided to purchase a van and fund a driver for the nursing home and ADCC but determined that ACCESS Transportation could meet the need to pick up and drop off clients. VCA used the nursing home's minivan for field trips and to take clients to appointments and therapy sessions.

In 1985, after almost three years of operation, ADCC achieved its first profit of $98.82 in revenue over expenses—though it continued to receive a $1,000 monthly subsidy from VCA. Grants from the Beaver County Office on Aging partially supported clients from Beaver County. The program also accepted Medicaid.

ELIZABETH G. MOORE SCHOLARSHIP FUND

VCA started the Elizabeth G. Moore Scholarship Fund in 1986 in honor of Betts Moore, director of development from 1981 until 1986. The funds gave some financial assistance to nursing home residents but primarily supported clients of the Adult Day Care Centers who could not afford the full fee on their own.

VCA members, client families, the Valley Care Auxiliary, the Staunton Farms Foundation, the Presbyterian Church of Sewickley and other charities donated money to the fund.

In 2003, the fund gave $12,000 in scholarships. In 2004, to bolster the fund, the Moore family gave $10,000, matching and exceeding $7,340 in donations raised from others. By 2011, the fund had $33,000.

Needy clients could receive 50 percent of their cost of care while they waited for county funding, not to exceed three months. That year, the VCA Adult Day Services (ADS) committee established new income parameters and criteria for using the funds.

In 2013, the fund was at $14,000 and decreasing due to increased requests from clients because of funding constraints at state and county levels. By 2018, the fund was no longer in existence, but ADS clients could request financial support through Lutheran SeniorLife.

MOVING TO AMBRIDGE

By 1986, the VCA ADCC was the fifth largest of the twenty-one day care centers in Allegheny County. It was beginning to outgrow its space in the Aleppo Township building.

In December 1986, the board raised client fees from twenty dollars to twenty-two dollars a day to cover the cost of meals and secretarial help. It also decided to move from Aleppo to Ambridge in Beaver County, Pennsylvania, about seven miles away. The program took over two rooms within the former school building of the Divine Redeemer Church at 233 Merchant Street in Ambridge.

The Ambridge ADCC was open from 8:00 a.m. to 5:00 p.m. on weekdays, and the daily fee included breakfast, lunch and a snack. Podiatry, dental and hairdressing services were available for a small fee.

In 1987, ADCC had eight clients from Allegheny County and twenty-three from Beaver County, reaching a new high of 256 client days in October. Most clients were on fixed incomes and could not afford day care without the subsidy, as attending for five days per week cost more than $500 per month.

FIVE-YEAR ANNIVERSARY

VCA hosted sixty-five guests at an open house to celebrate ADCC's five-year anniversary on June 10, 1988. At that point, service was provided to seventy-eight clients per week—the highest census ever. In fact, the facility had a waiting list for the limited number of spaces that were funded by grants from the Beaver County Office on Aging. At the same time, Allegheny County was supplying free transportation and food for its clients.

A creative art therapy program offered at the center in 1988 helped clients express their often-hidden feelings and emotions, if not on canvas then certainly on construction paper, according to Marsha Koschik, the new activities director at the center. Koschik had a Master of Science degree in art therapy with a specialization in geriatrics.[28] "Creative art therapy uses the

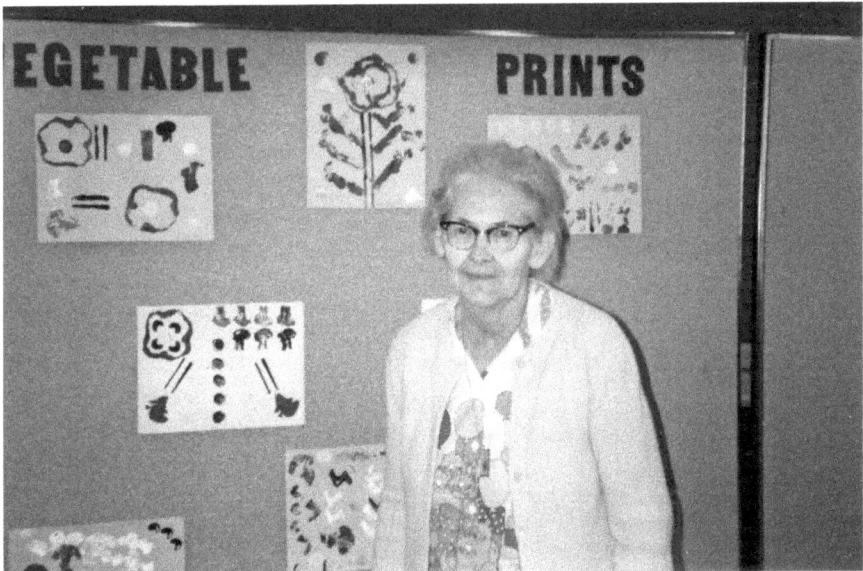

A proud ADCC client shows off the vegetable prints she created in 1995. *Courtesy of Valley Care Association.*

BOARD MEMBER PROFILE: GWEN OGLE

Gwen Ogle was Valley Care Auxiliary president and a VCA board member from 1991 until 2008. In 2010, she served a three-year term on the advisory council of the Allegheny County Area Agency on Aging. She said this about her experiences with her husband and Valley Care's ADCC:

There was Alzheimer's in my husband's family, so [when he developed symptoms] *I knew what it was about. I could see that I needed some help. So I took my husband, Jere, to the Adult Day Care in Ambridge. The people who work there treat each client as if he or she was their own grandparent.*

The staff let them do what they wanted to do, but kept them busy during the day. Jere was a neat freak, so he would get the broom out and clean up. That's what was important to him. It made him feel as if he was doing something important.

Family members often put up barriers that prevent them from seeking the help they need. Taking care of the person becomes their whole life. They don't want to relinquish the caregiver role. Part of that is the stigma caregivers seem to place on getting help. They also think that their family member wouldn't like to be in someone else's care, which is often not the case.

Because Jere was busy all day, I had time to run our business. Without Valley Care, I couldn't have done it. With it, we could stay together, at home, for another year and a half, until I had to move him to a nursing home.

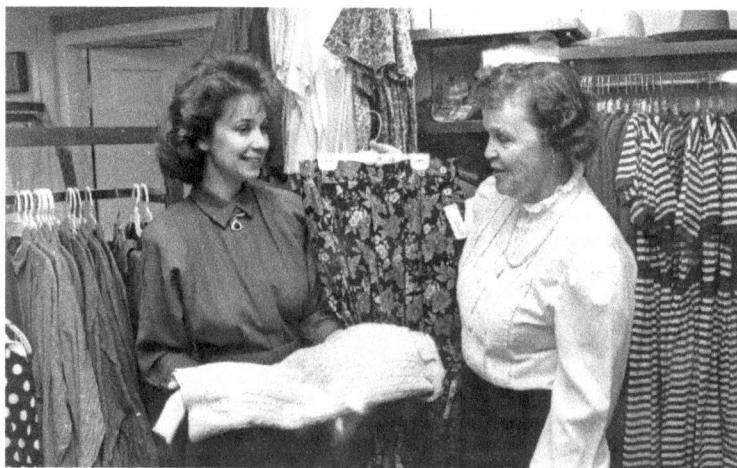

Gwen Ogle, president of VCA Auxiliary (*right*), prepares for a fashion show in 1992 with Lorraine Easton of Talbots clothing store. *Courtesy of Valley Care Association.*

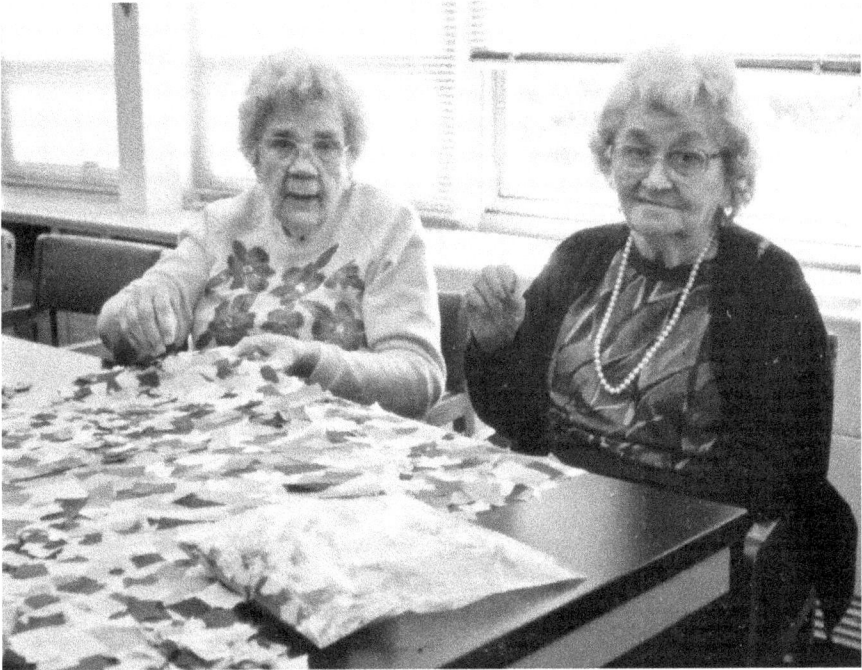

Two women working together on a collage at the ADCC in 1993. *Courtesy of Valley Care Association.*

concepts, tools, and techniques of the visual, musical, and performing arts in order to foster communication," she said.

With excess revenue over expenses and increasing client days, ADCC had been able to support itself during 1990. Based on this success, VCA decided to reward staff with a bonus of 10 percent of six months of salary when the staff to client ratio exceeded one to five and revenue exceeded expenses by established amounts. Several payouts were made over the coming years.

In 1991, ADCC increased the daily attendance by 13 percent, going from 3,565 client days to 4,035 client days. Revenues exceeded expense for the second consecutive year. That year, Allegheny and Beaver County Long-term Care Assessment and Management Program (LAMP) and the Pennsylvania Caregiver Program assisted families with the cost of care. Clients who needed financial assistance could also apply for scholarships from VCA's Elizabeth G. Moore Scholarship Fund.

TENTH ANNIVERSARY RECOGNIZED

As the ADCC marked its tenth anniversary in 1993, program participants were regularly engaged in friendly competition, playing basketball or bowling. They also interacted socially by dancing to piano music.

According to ADCC director James T. Ciocarello, activities were often based on the need to improve clients' communication and inter-relational skills.

George Haskell, a stroke survivor, went to the center four days a week, allowing his wife, Hilda, to do housework, play bridge or help out at her church. "He likes it here. He's with other people, where at home, he's just with me. It's wonderful for both of us," Hilda said.[29]

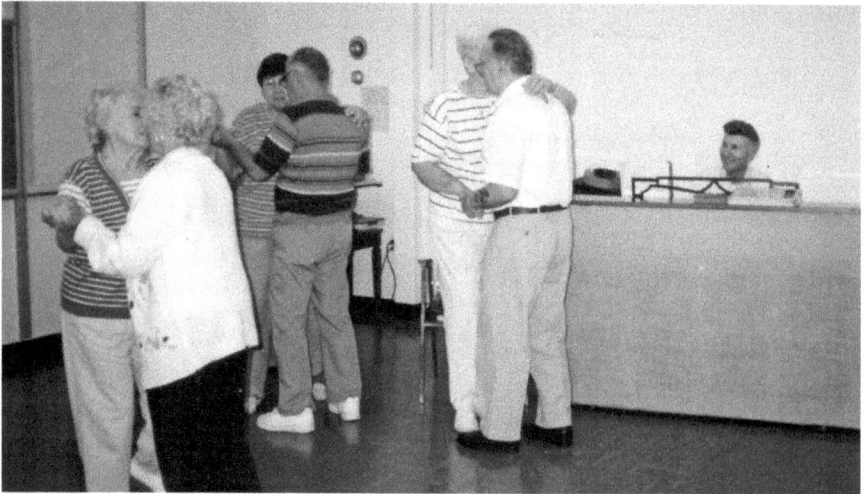

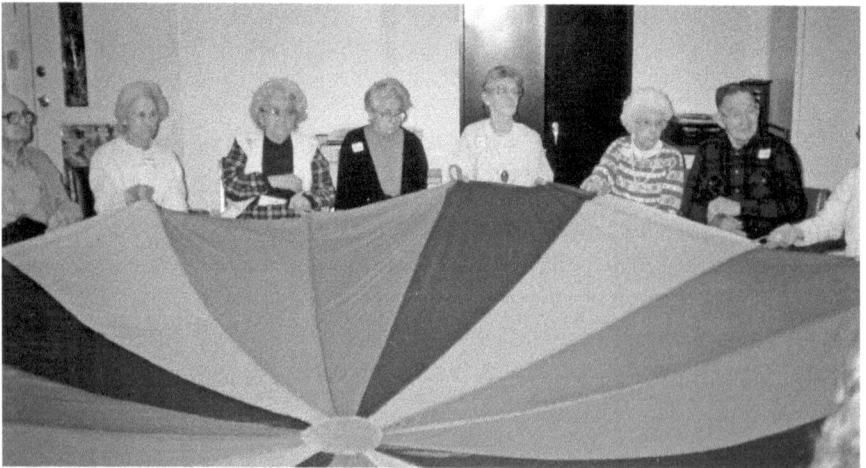

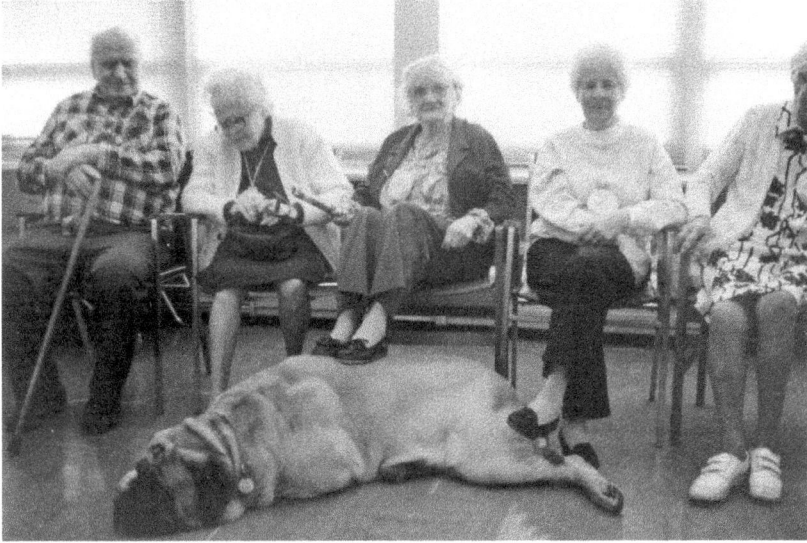

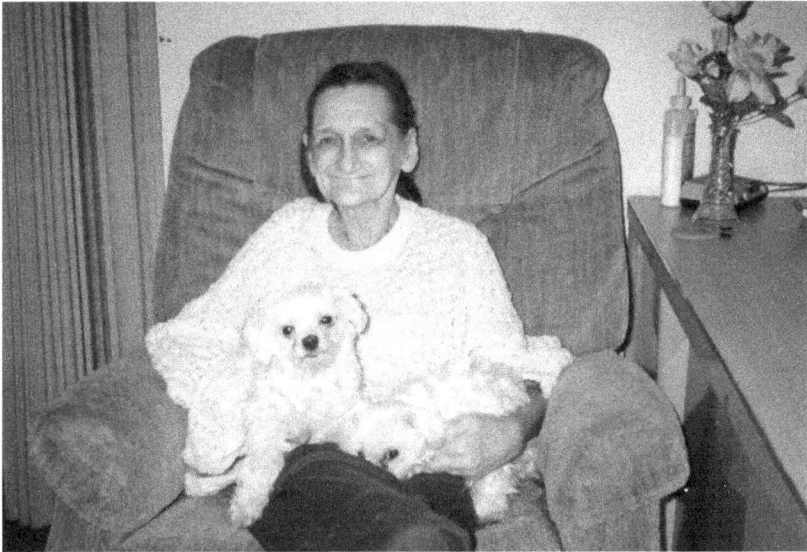

This page, top: Larger dogs were welcomed at pet therapy at the Ambridge ADCC in 1991. *Courtesy of Valley Care Association.*

This page, bottom: Pet therapy connected clients with their memories and reduced stress. *Courtesy of Valley Care Association.*

Opposite, top: Dancing to live music was a popular activity at the ADCC in 1997. *Courtesy of Valley Care Association.*

Opposite, bottom: Parachute physical therapy improved coordination at the ADCC in Ambridge, 1994. *Courtesy of Valley Care Association.*

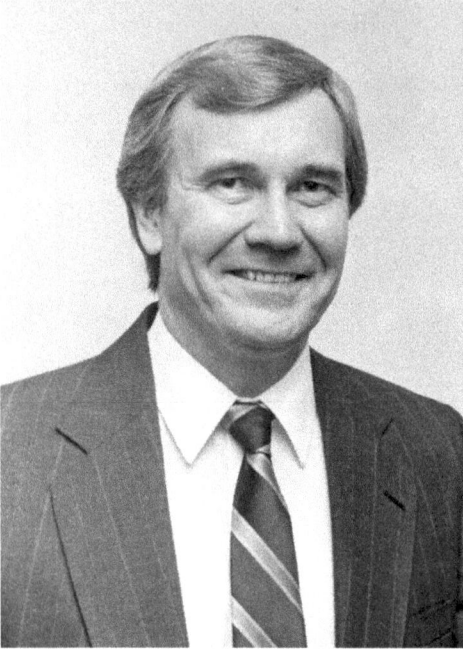

James Ciocarello, ADCC director, 1989–97. *Courtesy of Valley Care Association.*

Standard practices dictated a program that reinforced the mentally confused person's place in the "real world." Activities included exercise, current events, reality orientation, music and pet therapy, social interaction, games and arts and crafts designed to meet this goal.

Building a New Home in Ambridge

When the Catholic Diocese of Pittsburgh closed Divine Redeemer School in 1994, it granted the ADCC a month-to-month lease.

In 1995, the ADCC had a total of sixty-one clients. For the fifth straight year, the center achieved a 100 percent score for compliance in the Pennsylvania Department of Aging's annual survey. By 1996, the ADCC was serving fifty-nine clients, at fees of thirty-two dollars a day.

In 1999, after VCA sold the Valley Care Nursing Home to Masonic Village, it had money to improve the day care program and decided to invest in the construction of a new building for the ADCC. In 2000, VCA bought property at 325 Maplewood Avenue in Ambridge, which the Borough of Ambridge was selling for $7,000, and demolished the building on the site.

VCA also purchased an adjoining property from Holy Ghost Orthodox Church for $5,000 in May 2000. The combined space gave VCA more room on which to build a one-story, 3,100-square-foot facility at a cost of $497,000.

Designed by Lynch and Associates Architects of Pittsburgh, and built by R.E. Crawford Construction, the new center had a full-service therapeutic kitchen where clients could cook, a large central activity area, two small group activity rooms, a bathing area and a hairdresser sink. It could serve up to thirty-four clients with four full-time and three part-time workers.

Plans included an enclosed garden with a gazebo, raised planting beds and window boxes so that clients with physical limitations could participate. Paths were designed to be easy for those with Alzheimer's to navigate. Feeders and flowers attracted birds and butterflies.

Eight elderly clients wore hard hats and carried shovels for the groundbreaking ceremony on September 26, 2000. They were chauffeured in VCA's new fourteen-person van, which was bought through a $35,000 county grant.

Around that time, VCA changed the program's name to Adult Day Services (ADS). ADS provided a more structured program for clients with

---

CLIENT PROFILE: TED ZAJACKOWSKI

Janet Zajackowski brought her father, Ted, to Valley Care Adult Day Services in Ambridge and headed to work with confidence that her father was in very good hands until she returned at the end of her day.

"I could never feel comfortable going to work and leaving my dad at home alone all day," explained Janet. "At Valley Care he's with people who know him and I don't have to worry about anything."

Ted, eighty-eight, started attending Valley Care ADS in June 1995, six months after the death of his wife. When his daughter took over as his full-time caregiver, she needed a solution that would allow her to work yet enable her father to continue to live at home.

"If it was not for Valley Care Adult Day Services, I would have had to place him in a nursing home," stated Janet. "He does not like to be alone, and he needs someone to keep him company almost all of the time. It's so nice to have the people at Valley Care who can be with him when I am not able." *

---

* VCA Annual Report, 1998–99.

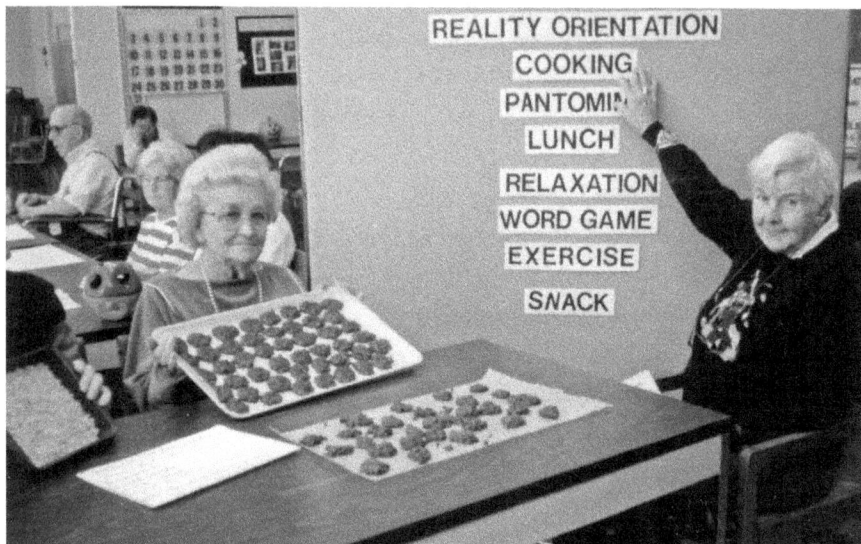

Baking cookies was one of the activities used to stimulate mental health in 1993 at the ADCC. *Courtesy of Valley Care Association.*

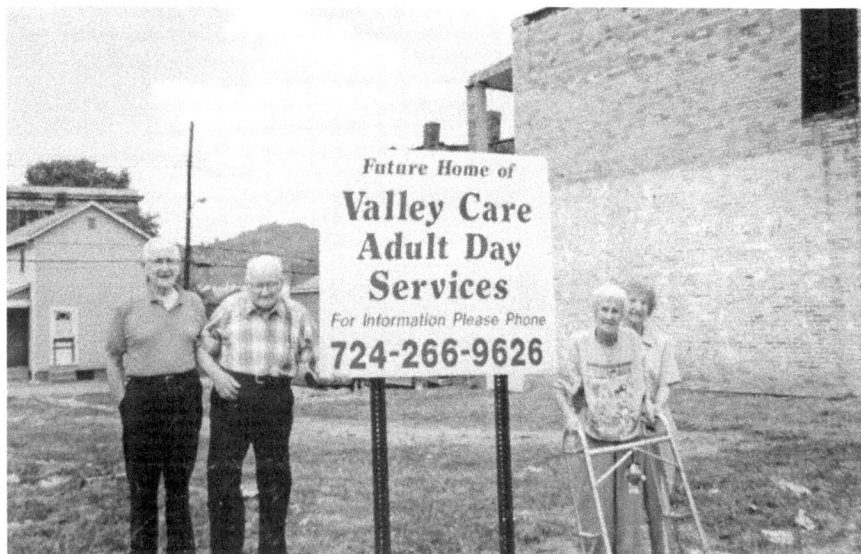

In 2000, ADCC clients John Morris, Ted Zajaczkowski, Catherine Kokoski and Eleanor Yovanovic stand on the ADCC building site in Ambridge. *Courtesy of Valley Care Association.*

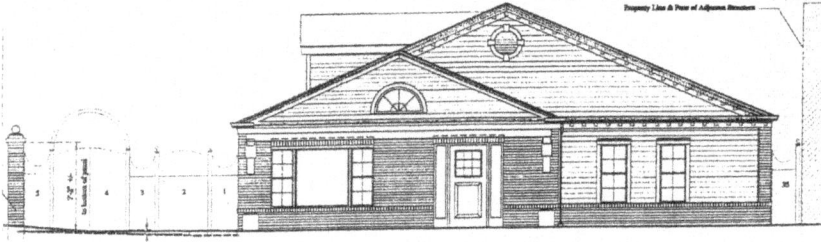

Adult Day Care Facility
345 Maplewood Avenue   Ambridge   Beaver County   PA

Valley Care Association
400 Broad Street   Sewickley   Allegheny County   Pennsylvania

Lynch and Associates Architects of Pittsburgh drew this rendering of the new ADCC on Maplewood Avenue in Ambridge in 2000. *Courtesy of Valley Care Association.*

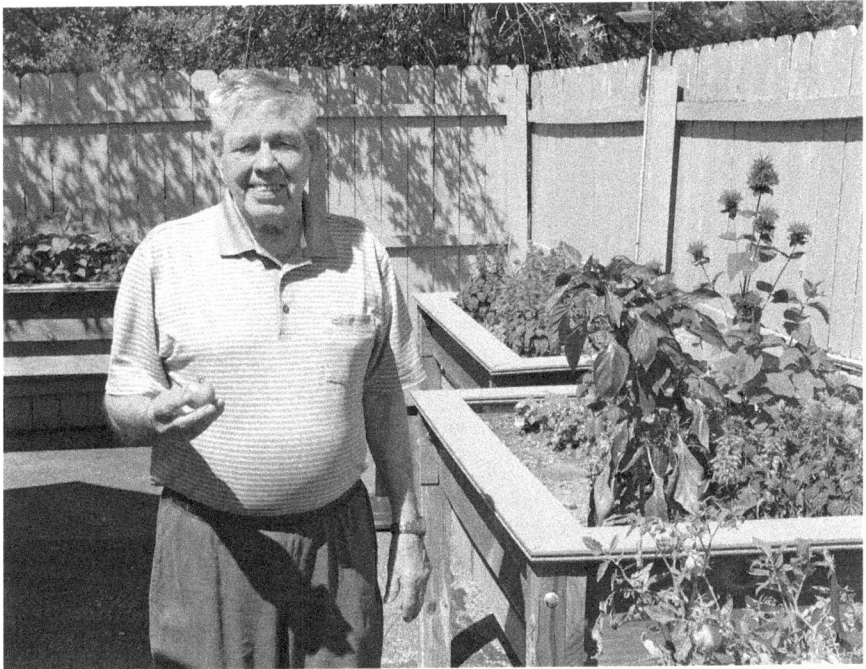

Seniors tended the outdoor garden at the ADCC in Ambridge through 2018. *Courtesy of Valley Care Association.*

BOARD MEMBER PROFILE: DAN PETERS

Dan Peters of Moon Township served on the VCA board from 2003 until 2012, focusing on financial matters and assuming the presidency in 2008. In discussing VCA, he said:

> When I came onboard in 2003, the primary focus was the ADS. VCA had come into a large sum of money as the result of the sale of the [nursing home] property, and our objective was to preserve the windfall and see what good things we could do with it. Primarily, to support the ADS operations in Ambridge and Moon.
>
>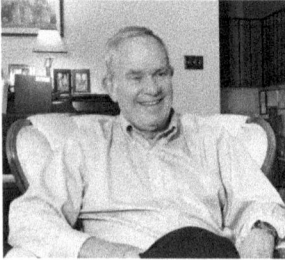
>
> There were some older adults with physical issues and mental acuity, and others with dementia and mental disabilities. It was hard to do the same program for both groups. A lot of administrators were needed to do both.
>
> Of course, there were some disappointments. But it was very satisfying to get accolades from the caregivers and families. They were always very pleased with the service.

Dan Peters. *Courtesy of Mark Grover, Mark Ten Productions.*

Alzheimer's and other severe memory impairments. With a grant of $5,000 from the Pittsburgh National Bank Charitable Trust, VCA created a separate room for these clients that was more secure and tailored to their needs with therapeutic activities designed to ease the frustration and depression that accompany the condition.

"When we built the place in Ambridge, we designed the rooms to be very homey," said Ogle. "So the elderly would feel like it was home, what they were used to." The new center opened on April 2, 2001, with a census split evenly between Allegheny and Beaver counties and plans to increase visibility in Allegheny County.

CARING FOR THE CONFUSED AND DISORIENTED

Deb Shtulman was executive director of VCA from 2001 until 2008. She felt that the stigma and denial surrounding Alzheimer's disease was part of the reason day care centers weren't more popular.

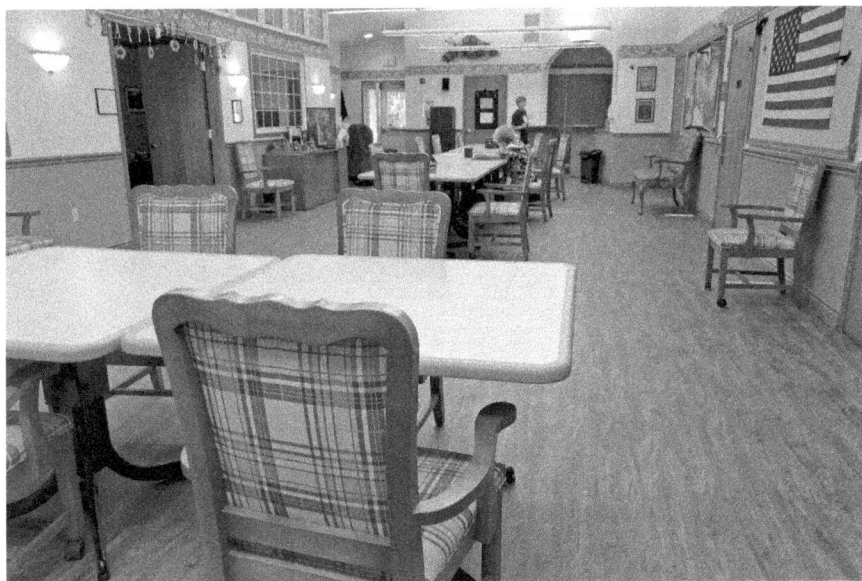

The main activity room at the Ambridge ADCC was built in 2017. *Courtesy of Valley Care Association.*

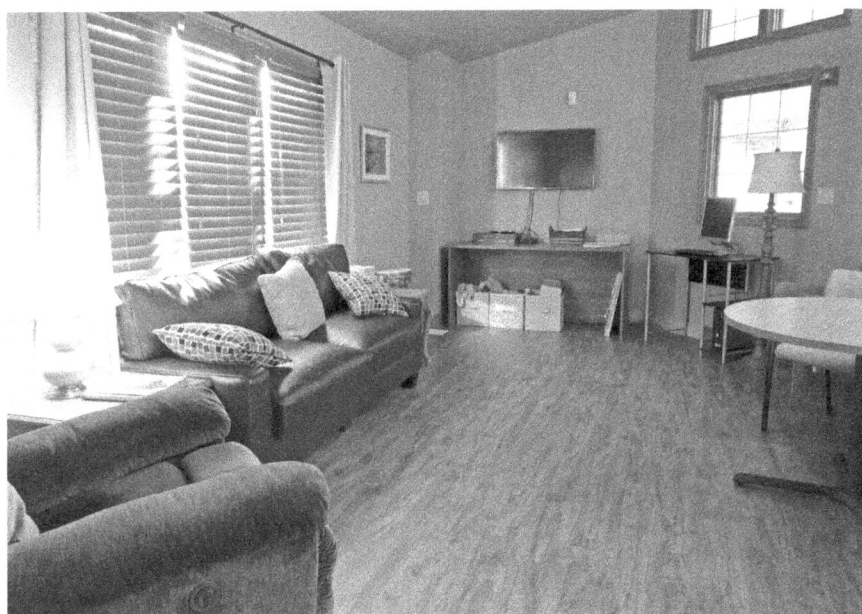

Off the main activity room of the Ambridge ADCC, this smaller room was used for one-on-one activities and medical care. *Courtesy of Valley Care Association.*

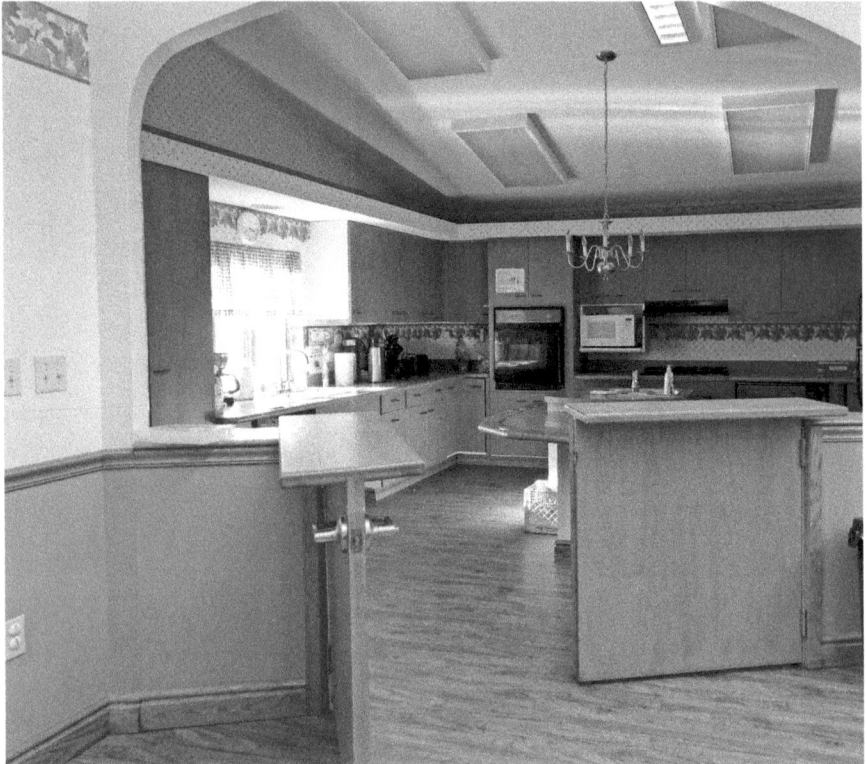

Completed in 2017, the new Ambridge ADCC had a modern kitchen. *Courtesy of Valley Care Association.*

"Once families became part of our community, they would often ask themselves, 'Why didn't we do this sooner?'" she said. "When someone develops dementia, they hide the memory loss. The family is in crisis. They tell me that we won't understand their mom, or she doesn't want to come, or that she's not bad enough yet."

During these years, more clients arrived after having a stroke, heart attack or chronic disease. Others showed a greater mental decline, which limited their activities.

As for those with dementia, Shtulman explained that it took a great amount of effort to care for these patients. "Of course, it took longer for the staff to get to know people who were more fully along in the progression of disease. Especially if they came only once a week. For them, every week was new. But once they came in, their families were relieved. The clients had a full day and were tired, ready to go home," she said.

"I don't know how the staff did it," Ogle said. "No arguments, no yelling, and no clients on medication either. Diabetics got their insulin. Others got meals, showers, and personal care. All these things were very helpful to the family. If you want to relate to people with dementia, you have to get into their world, because they are never coming into yours."

NEXT STEPS IN SERVICES

In 2003, all county day care clients were asked to pay a share of their costs that had previously been covered by the Allegheny or Beaver County Area Agency on Aging. This change caused many adult day service sites in Allegheny County to shut down. Others experienced 30 to 50 percent declines in clients over eighteen months.

In response, adult day service providers in Allegheny County formed a coalition—the ADS Network Center for Daytime Living—to target marketing to private pay clients, especially those with annual earnings of more than $40,000. The goal was to relieve caregivers' burdens and increase client satisfaction.

At its tactical planning retreat in 2004, the VCA board determined that "without Adult Day Services, VCA really doesn't have any tangible purpose." Ideally, VCA wanted to spend 10 percent on ADS and 90 percent on grants. Instead, VCA was spending 80 percent of its resources on ADS and 20 percent on grants, which was not sustainable in the long term.

CLIENT PROFILE: HELEN

Helen attended Valley Care Adult Day Services starting in 1997, when she was diagnosed with Alzheimer's disease. Her doctor recommended adult day services to provide social stimulation and medical oversight for Helen and respite for her daughter and primary caregiver, Patty.

"I am so grateful that there is a place where my mother can enjoy activities and friends. Adult day services are good for the person and good for the family," Patty said. "If you are with your family member 24 hours a day, you have no life. This is the best thing for both of us. When she comes home at the end of the day, Mom is happy."[*]

---

[*] VCA Annual Report, 2003.

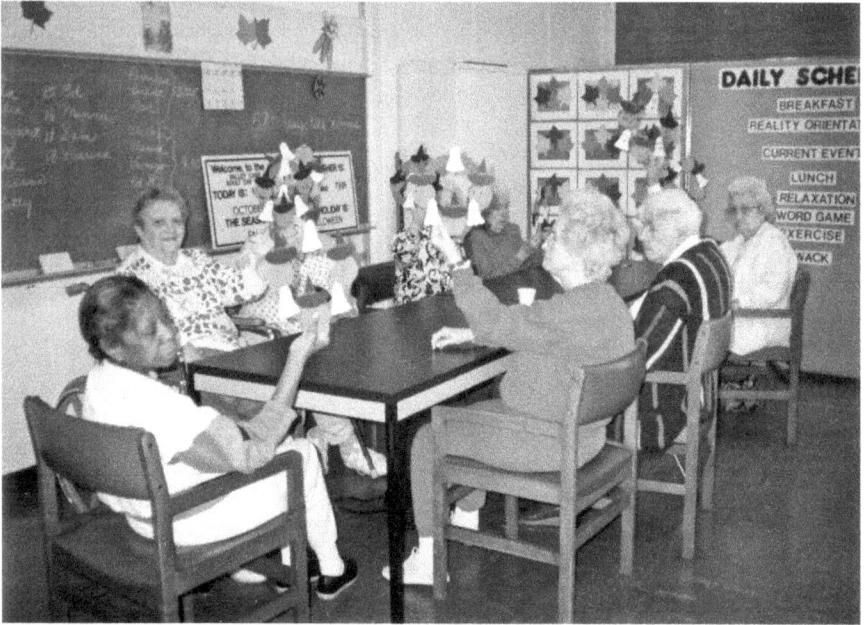

Above: In October 1993, ADCC clients create seasonal crafts. *Courtesy of Valley Care Association.*

Left: Socialization and friendships were important factors to maintain good mental health at the ADCC in 1996. *Courtesy of Valley Care Association.*

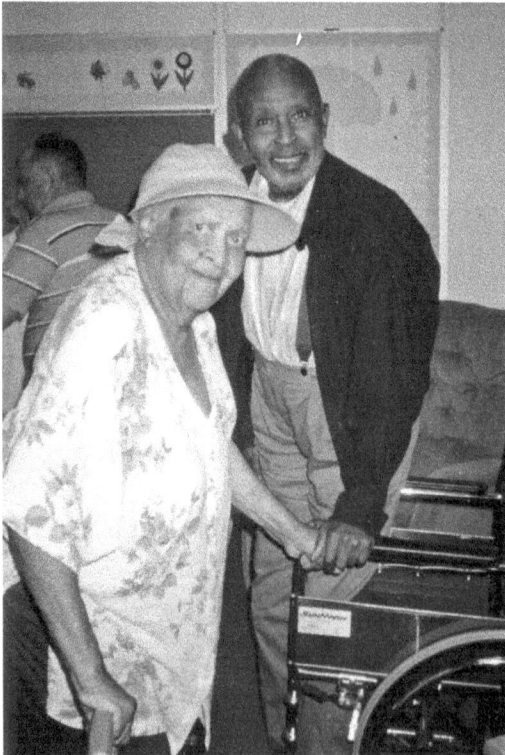

To improve the viability of ADS, the board considered updated programming, increased revenue from outside sources, third party payers, marketing efforts and the use of the building for community programs. It also decided to explore the private market, other revenue streams or even selling the service to another social service organization.

AN UPSWING IN ATTENDANCE

In 2005, a $1.6 billion deficit in the Pennsylvania Medicaid program pushed clients to home- and community-based services. Medicaid introduced its Community Choice Initiative, a program designed to reduce the wait between referral and service delivery from six weeks to forty-eight hours. It had the potential to increase referrals, starting in 2006.

This program may have been a factor in the growth of Valley Care's ADS census, which finished the year with net income of $1,058 instead of the projected $45,587 loss. Bolstered by these positive results, ADS considered a respite program for people caring for elderly at home that would offer overnight and daytime care.

By the end of the year, with a daily census of twenty-eight, ADS had a waiting list of five people. It added staff and sought more volunteers. Fifty nursing students from Sewickley Valley Hospital and two from Duquesne University in Pittsburgh came to the center as part of their nursing curriculum, gaining valuable skills while helping clients.

In 2006, Medicare conducted a project to study the idea of delivering a portion of a patient's home health services within medical adult day care facilities. The hope was that it could reduce Medicare costs. The study showed that only 12 percent of home care patients who attended adult day services as part of their plan of care were readmitted to the hospital, compared with 28.8 percent of home care patients who did not receive adult day services.

EXPANDING ACROSS THE RIVER

In 2007, VCA began looking into building another facility to accommodate the people on its waiting list and focused on Moon Township. The first location considered was on Beaver Grade Road. The second was at 650 Cherrington Boulevard, in an industrial park with many office buildings.

The second location was chosen for several reasons, including:

- A capacity for fifty clients, with a target of sixteen per day
- A lease of $55,000
- A $340,000 budget for Thomas Construction to build out the site
- Eight clients who were interested in moving there
- Nearby businesses might be interested in offering day care as an employee benefit
- A cost of seventy dollars per day compared to Ambridge at sixty-two dollars per day

"We chose an office park with older workers, people who were supporting their parents and giving care to them. It was a great thought process, but the market wasn't there," said Peters. "We contacted the human resources departments of local companies in the office park and offered them ADS as a local service, as a potential benefit to their employees."

The Cherrington ADS opened during the summer of 2009, with a site manager and program coordinator, nurse and program assistant, as well as a short-term, part-time marketing consultant. Twelve clients transferred from Ambridge.

VCA added a full-time marketing position to promote how ADS struck a balance between managing clients' medical needs and maintaining the environment of a "social club." Occupational therapy students from the University of Pittsburgh enriched their studies by working with seniors in a very practical, hands-on way at both ADS sites.

VCA continued to explore options that would better serve clients, some of which had short-term success and others that never went beyond the discussion stage:

- Extending the day to eleven hours in Ambridge
- Offering a six-hour, partial-day session at Moon
- Hosting a date night for couples living with dementia
- Offering services to the under-sixty population

In 2011, marketing efforts were in full swing, including a St. Patrick's Day open house, a monthly caregiver support group and a diabetes disease management workshop. VCA contacted businesses, churches and health care providers. To encourage referrals, ADS joined the Sewickley Ministerium group and strengthened its relationship with Faith in Action, a program of the Sewickley Valley YMCA.

CLIENT PROFILE: RICK JAMISON

Rick Jamison, only fifty-two years old, had a chronic medical condition leading to confusion and anxiety, as well as physical impairment. Rick was married to his wife, Barbara, for more than twenty-five years and had been very active for most of those years as an avid hunter and fisherman. As his illness progressed, Barb noticed a marked difference in Rick's ability to care for himself while she was at work.

A friend suggested she look into adult day services to reduce her level of concern about Rick while she was away from home. Valley Care became Rick's safe harbor. He settled into the routine, and Barbara informed the staff, "I cannot say enough good things about this place. I know I don't have to worry about Rick while I am at work."[*]

---

[*] VCA Annual Report, 2000.

VOLUNTEERS PLAY A VITAL ROLE

Volunteers were always an important part of the ADS program. They provided a new point of contact to stimulate clients—and someone new to hear their stories. Volunteers shared their creative talents, teaching cooking, woodworking or crafts, and provided extra supervisory skills and helping hands, especially during outings.

Alan Miliner volunteered because his mother, Anna, was a client at ADS. When she passed away, he spent his vacation volunteering in Ambridge. "Helping out at the center has helped me with the grieving process," Miliner said. "Especially around the holidays. I didn't want to sit around and dwell on things. Doing something for someone else keeps me from doing that." He helped with lunch, bingo, the annual holiday party and outings.[30]

Louis Gilberti started volunteering after his wife enrolled as a client in Moon Township. He accompanied the clients on field trips to a pumpkin patch hayride and an afternoon of bowling. He danced a polka with a ninety-five-year-old client at Robin Hill Park. "I like helping out," said Gilberti. "The people here are nice, and I enjoy getting to know the clients and staff."[31]

STRIVING TO REMAIN SUSTAINABLE

In 2012, VCA found itself at a crossroads. Ongoing subsidies to ADS would eventually drain VCA's financial resources. It was essential to find a way to make these programs self-sustaining within the next two to three years. The alternative was to find a company that might wish to invest in the organization.

VCA was not alone. At least 50 percent of adult day care centers in the region were not doing well, and five planned to close. In exploring options, VCA applied for a $1 million Innovation Challenge from the Centers for

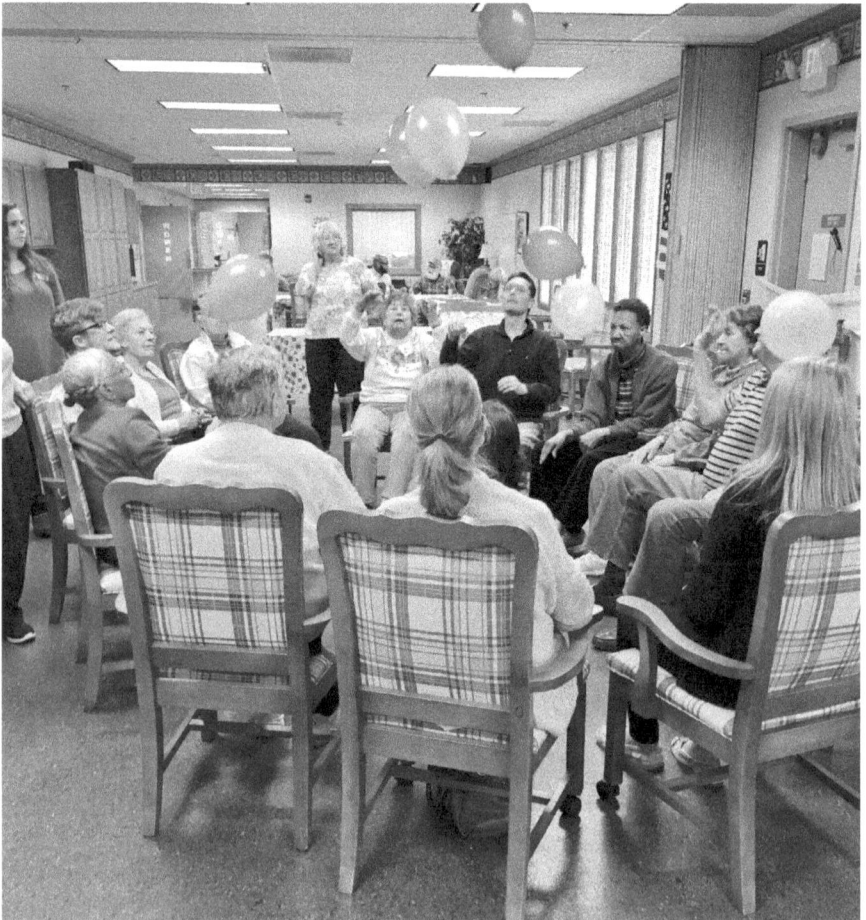

In 2018, clients of ADS in Moon Township maintained their physical health with games and activities. *Courtesy of Valley Care Association.*

Medicare and Medicaid Service (CMS) to create a post-acute rehabilitation model that could lower the costs of rehabilitation after hospital care. Though VCA did not receive the grant, it continued to seek other ways to offer ADS as a temporary transitional care option for certain hospital discharges.

Susan Nirschel, RN, was hired as the new director of the Moon and Ambridge sites in March 2012, and a new client services specialist position was introduced. With this restructuring, the board also considered expanding the populations served to include those under age sixty and with various diagnoses; offering additional services, such as transportation; changing the fee schedule and minimum attendance requirement; and retaining an occupational therapist to evaluate the impact of ADS on health.

VCA adopted a new vision statement in anticipation of these changes: "We empower individuals and caregivers of all ages to be active, safe, and healthy."

Despite the changes and increased options, a large part of VCA's revenue was not from the ADS. About 42 percent of VCA's revenue continued to come from the VCA endowment and investment portfolio.

PARTNERING WITH LUTHERAN SENIORLIFE

In the fall of 2012, VCA's executive committee met with Lutheran SeniorLife (LSL), an organization committed to rebranding care for the elderly that operated in Beaver, Armstrong, Lawrence, Butler and Allegheny Counties.

The missions of the two organizations were aligned. VCA hoped that working with LSL would allow VCA to preserve its endowment and keep its programs viable. Following a presentation by LSL president and CEO David Fenoglietto in December 2012, the VCA board approved and authorized formal discussions with LSL.

"VCA needed to partner with someone to keep this venture alive," said Eric Gross, executive director of Masonic Village and VCA board president. "LSL had a stake in keeping people out of nursing homes, and could help the ADS with transportation, employees, clients, and office space."

Discussions with LSL continued in 2013 as the two organizations strived to establish a business relationship that would combine their strengths to benefit the elderly in the region. During negotiations, LSL was concerned about the financial burden the affiliation was going to place on its organization.

Eventually, a nonbinding letter of intent gave LSL managerial control of Valley Care ADS.

Valley Care Endowment, which distributed funds for VCA, would:

- Continue to financially support the ADS for three years, up to agreed-upon monetary limits
- Provide additional support in years four and five
- Maintain the corpus of its investment at no less than $5 million

The affiliation agreement was signed on August 20, 2013, giving LSL management responsibility for and financial revenues from the two ADS facilities. VCA retained the ADS, including the property and building it owned in Ambridge. Steps had been taken to anticipate the new arrangement:

- VCA closed its corporate office in Sewickley on June 14, 2013, a significant and symbolic shift in the history of the organization.

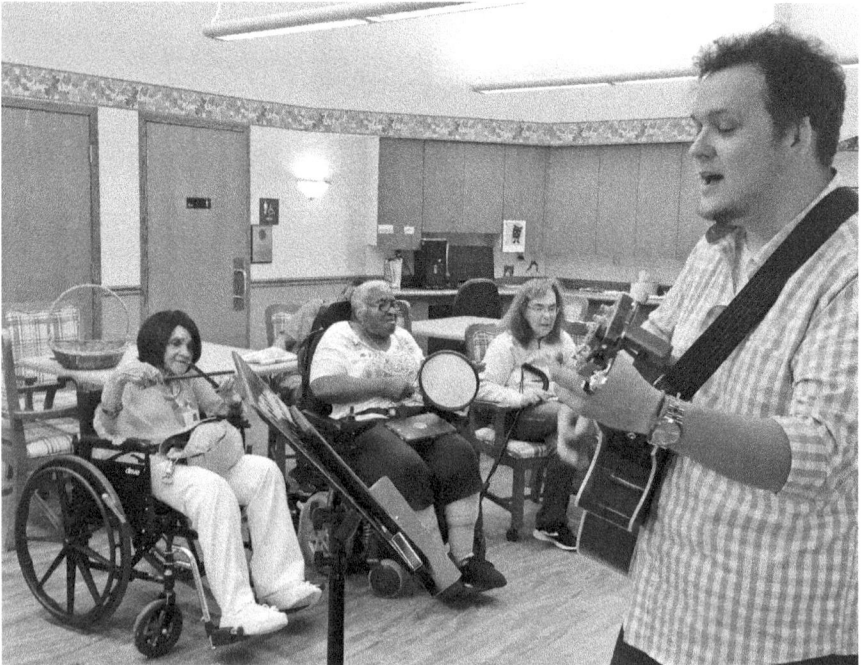

Managed by Lutheran SeniorLife, the ADS continued to emphasize socialization through music, which brings back memories for older adults. *Courtesy of Valley Care Association.*

- The executive director functions were split between Susan Nirschel, director of ADS, and Toni Hively, executive director of LSL's LIFE program (Living Independently for the Elderly) that helped older adults stay in their homes.
- Staffing and upkeep were split between VCA and LIFE Beaver.
- Administrative staff members relocated to the Moon and Ambridge ADS sites.

Building on its previous experience, LSL reduced the operating cost of the ADS sites by consolidating staff and management services, as well as purchasing supplies and services for the entire organization. LSL also applied the experience and expertise from across its wide network.

From 2013 to 2018, LSL received financial support from VCE but assumed the costs, received the revenue, managed the day-to-day operations, cared for residents, hired employees and did all marketing and administrative services.

"By aligning with LSL, we could achieve significant economies of scale and management efficiency," said Brooks. "This allowed us to control costs, but the question of how to grow our volume still remained. Revenues did not grow to the point where ADS could be self-sustaining."

8

Supporting the Community
through Grants, 1999–Present

We will be awarding grants to projects that enhance the quality of life for older adults in [the] community...and promote aging at home as a safer, more realistic choice.
—*Jane Ellen Tumpson, VCA executive director*

With $8 million in proceeds from the sale of the Valley Care Nursing Home to the Masons in 1999, Valley Care Association (VCA) had an unanticipated opportunity to serve the senior community in new ways.

The board considered starting a number of programs to serve seniors, including transportation services, respite care, telephone reassurance, adult resources, information and referral services, hospice care, caregiver training, homemaker services, maintenance, scholarship subsidies and a new Adult Day Services site—possibly in Sewickley.

Ultimately, the board decided against entering into another direct-care operation and instead agreed to start a foundation and fulfill its mission by providing financial support to outside organizations focused on services for seniors. In this way, VCA felt it could use the money as the original donors had intended.

In the 1998–99 annual report, VCA president James Alexander stated, "I am proud to be involved in the formation of a new vision for Valley Care. The prospects for facilitating the provision of many services and programs for older adults are limitless. We will work collaboratively with a number of like-minded organizations and are thrilled to have the financial resources to support the activities so clearly needed to add to the quality of life for aging adults in the Sewickley Valley region."

VCA invested the monies gained through the sale of the nursing home and actively supported nonprofit projects that advanced its mission. "We will manage those investments and further the VCA's charitable purpose by serving as a foundation," said VCA executive director Jane Ellen Tumpson. "[We will be] awarding grants to projects which enhance the quality of life for older adults in [the] community and which promote aging at home as a safer, more realistic choice." The goal was to award at least five grants during fiscal year 1999–2000.

VCA also developed collaborative relationships with other community organizations and continued to provide financial support to the ADS program, which was not self-supporting.

TWO NEW COMMITTEES SUPPORT GRANT PROGRAM

VCA created a grants committee to establish a clearly defined application procedure and approval process that included program goals, grant-making strategies and funding priorities. The committee determined that the amount awarded would vary each year, depending on the needs of the community and the performance of the VCA investment portfolio.

To help publicize the new grants program and learn about the needs of Sewickley and the surrounding communities, VCA also created an ad hoc community liaison committee. This committee organized and hosted town meetings in the winter and spring of 2000–01 in Ambridge, Moon/Coraopolis, Sewickley and Aliquippa. It presented VCA's new goals and plans and asked about the needs of seniors in each town.

The meetings revealed similar needs in all the communities: transportation, information and referral, home safety and maintenance and care in the community (respite, home care and supportive services).

VCA set grant-making goals and responsibilities for programs:

- Serve older people with limited incomes or no government or family support
- Advocate for older adults who didn't have a voice
- Build understanding among ethnic, racial and generation groups in the community
- Create safe places for the elderly to live
- Support a long-term commitment to seniors in the area

BOARD MEMBER PROFILE: DANIEL H. BROOKS, MD

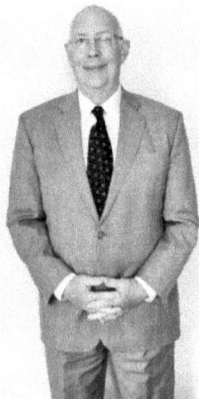

Daniel H. Brooks, MD.
Courtesy of Valley Care Association.

Dan Brooks, MD, joined the Valley Care Association Board in 2008 and served as president in 2012. He moved to the Valley Care Endowment Board in 2014.

"The Valley Care Board members followed a compulsive organizational and documentation process that allowed them to develop a comprehensive view of what it takes to establish a community-based, bodacious enterprise," said Brooks. "This planning process was led by experienced consultants who set forth specific and objective realistic implementation plans and demonstrated principles that any community-based entity should utilize."

Brooks came to Sewickley in 1978 as a physician with Surgical Associates of Sewickley. He treated hundreds of local people at his office and at their homes, because he believed that getting to know his patients' families and their personal circumstances was an essential part of patient care.

Brooks retired from private practice in 2000 to become chief medical officer for Heritage Valley Health System. He also served as its vice president for physician practices. He was chief operating officer of Sewickley Valley Hospital and vice president of community health services for Heritage Valley.

In 2013, the Allegheny County Medical Society (ACMS) gave Brooks its Richard E. Deitrick Humanity in Medicine award, which honors a physician who has improved the lives of patients and served as a role model for other physicians.

Brooks follows elder-care issues regionally and nationally and is interested in studying and developing community-based programs designed to address the social determinants of health and wellness. He is on the board of the ACMS Foundation, which supports healthy children and families in Allegheny County.

GUIDELINES FOR ELIGIBLE PROPOSALS

The grant-making guidelines were reviewed several times over the years, always with a focus on supporting the VCA mission. Applications were received either through a call for proposals to address a specific problem or through unsolicited project proposals that were received and evaluated throughout the year. Preference was given to applicants affiliated with public agencies or who were tax-exempt 501(c)(3) agencies.

VCA was very clear on the types of projects and expenses it would *not* fund: ongoing general operating expenses or existing deficits, endowment funds, basic biomedical research, research on drug therapies or devices, international programs and institutions, direct support of individuals and lobbying of any kind. Grants were rarely given to fund conferences or publications, but exceptions were made for opportunities that supported the VCA mission.

Within the acceptable areas of funding, VCA established three priorities for its grants:

- Unstable health conditions
- Healthy living
- Improved access to health and social services

CONSIDERING APPLICATIONS

Organizations interested in applying for grants had to complete grant proposals that included a brief description of the problem to be tackled, including justification of need, and a description of the proposed project, principal objectives and expected outcomes, as well as components or methodology, a timetable, how results were to be measured and distributed and risks and limitations. In addition, applicants had to have a budget, including income, expenses and other funding sources, and qualifications of the organization and staff to implement the project.

The first requests came from Union Aid Society, Adult Resources and Valley Care Masonic Center. VCA also committed to ongoing financial support to Valley Care's own ADS.

Grant requests were handled on a rolling review basis with the goal of three granting cycles per year. Initially, the grants committee established several criteria to apply to all grants:

- Grants to be awarded up to $20,000
- Multi-year grants to help establish programs were not to exceed three years
- With the exception of multi-year grants, organizations could not receive a second grant within one year to prevent VCA from becoming the sole funder

In March 2000, the first grants were awarded to:

- Valley Care Masonic Center: $10,000 for production and distribution of a senior services referral directory
- Generations Together: $25,963 (up to $33,463) to fund five intergenerational programs in the Sewickley Valley area for $1,500 each and $18,500 for technical assistance

A total of $106,000 in grants was awarded in the first year, 1999–2000.

Over the years, a number of organizations, such as the *Beaver County Senior News*, Project for Love and Faith in Action, received multiple grants. Grant recipients were required to submit annual progress reports on the use of the funds and the success of their funded programs. VCA requested the return of unused funds from organizations that were not successful in their missions.

By the end of 2001, more than $200,000 in additional grants were awarded, totaling $322,262. A full list of organizations that received grants is included in the appendix.

Grassroots Grants

One example of a grant that helped a small community group make a difference was Project for Love. Project for Love was a "sewing circle at the Leetsdale senior high-rise apartments that made pillows for hospital patients," said board member Dan Peters. "These were elderly women who liked to sew, so we helped them buy material."

Deb Shtulman, VCA executive director, also remembered the group. "They made blankets and hats for babies at the hospital," she said. "It was one of many programs in the community that gave the elderly opportunities for socializing together and enriching their lives as well."

Funding Programs to Keep Seniors Independent

Faith in Action

Faith in Action, a program of the Sewickley Valley YMCA, trained volunteers from local congregations to visit, provide transportation and do light housekeeping to alleviate the loneliness and frustration of advancing age. Faith in Action volunteers provided 8,265 hours of service in 2003–2004. The program was still active in 2018, when it had sixty-five drivers making 55,000 trips a year, taking older adults to the doctor or on other errands.

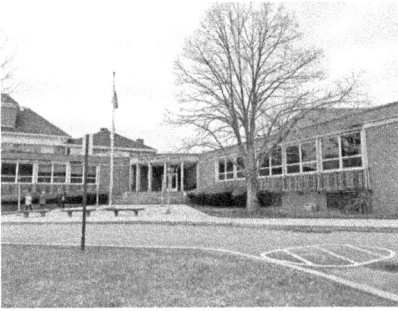

VCA awarded grants to the Sewickley YMCA for Faith in Action. *Courtesy of Valley Care Association.*

VCA awarded grants to the organization in 2003, 2004 and 2005. In 2004, VCA sponsored the River City Brass Band Holiday Concert at the Sewickley United Methodist Church, a holiday tradition that lasted several years and raised additional funds for Faith in Action.

Western Regional Wisdom Center

In 2004 and 2005, VCA funded the Western Regional Wisdom Center, a program of the Lutheran Service Society of Western Pennsylvania and its partner agencies. It offered seniors wellness services and lifelong learning. The program addressed physical, social, intellectual and emotional wellness. It also offered volunteer activities that encouraged participants to pass their skills and knowledge to the younger generation.

Over Eighty Initiative

In 2002, the Over Eighty Initiative received a grant from VCA. As Heritage Valley Health System's Community Case Management program, it assisted those older than age eighty to be independent through home visits from nurses and social workers. Support continued in 2003 when it served one hundred seniors.

Financial Downturn Affects Grants

There were periods when no grants were made due to market conditions and performance of the investment portfolio. Early in VCA's grant-making program, the United States experienced a recession. The result was an unrealized loss in the organization's investment portfolio of nearly $2 million over two years, all but stopping grants in 2001 and 2002.

"The $2 million loss paralyzed our grant making strategy," said Dan Brooks. "Coupled with the capital expenses of more than $1 million to operate the Adult Day Services, it truly diminished the power of the endowment. The final factor was the progressive deficits in the ADS programs, which required ongoing substantial contributions from VCA/VCE to stay afloat. Ultimately, we became mired in our own operational losses."

VCE's contribution to support VCA Adult Day Services was $500,000 a year from 2007 to 2013. The payment was capped at $375,000 for fiscal year 2014–2015 after Lutheran SeniorLife took over management of ADS. When LSL was able to reduce operating expenses, the contribution was cut to $225,000 from 2016 to 2018. VCA continued to own the centers as physical assets.

No grant approvals were recorded in the minutes after 2012. However, in October 2018, the board approved a grant of $2,300 to enable the Sewickley YMCA's Faith in Action program to purchase computer software to schedule volunteer drivers online and match them with older adults who needed transportation.

Home Safe Home, 1997–Present

*Helping to identify and correct safety hazards so that you can continue to live
independently and safely in your own home.*
—2006 Home Safe Home brochure

Addressing Safety at Home

The goal for many seniors—and their families—is to remain at home. One of the obvious critical factors to remaining at home is having a safe home in which to live. In fact, home safety was cited as a major concern in town hall meetings conducted by Valley Care Association (VCA) in 1999. VCA would play an active role in helping to make seniors' homes more livable through Home Safe Home (HSH), a program it operated from 2002 until 2014.

HSH was founded in 1997 by the Sewickley Valley Hospital (SVH) and ElderCare Coalition, a local group of gerontology professionals in the western suburbs of Pittsburgh. Adopted by the United Way of Allegheny County, the program was offered throughout the county with services that aligned with VCA's mission to serve seniors.

Over the years, HSH services expanded and were provided at three levels: distribution of "Home Safety Self Evaluation" booklets, home safety inspections and installations. Volunteers did free home evaluations to identify safety hazards and provided education to avoid accidents, distributing free bathmats, smoke detectors and nightlights.

They made minor home repairs and recommended more serious repairs when necessary, providing bids from independent contractors and handymen who were screened and fully insured. Funding was provided by government agencies, grants, corporations and private donations. The program was popular, often operating at capacity but also under a financial deficit.

Adult Resources, a Coraopolis senior services non-profit, assumed responsibility for the service in 1999 and, in 2000, requested funding from VCA's grant program. Though VCA questioned Adult Resources' ability to administer the program, VCA awarded funding for two years with the potential for a third year.

With the funding, Adult Resources redesigned the program to provide a self-help safety guide to all area residents. The new focus also included direct home safety services, such as installing bathroom grab bars, interior and exterior stair railings and wheelchair ramps.

In April 2001, John Seitz joined HSH as part-time program coordinator, working two days a week. An artist and art director with a degree in social work, Seitz had decided to leave his career and go back to school to take sociology classes in gerontology.

ADVERTISING FLYER FOR HOME SAFE HOME

Home Safe Home can help you with all your home safety concerns from a small fix-it job to a major home modification. We have the knowledge and experience to make your home a safer home, and as we are a nonprofit organization, your cost will be reasonable or subsidized through our financial assistance grants.

Home Safe Home can also provide:

· A free self-guided home safety workbook so you can check the safety of your home.
· A safety professional who will walk through your home with you to identify any safety hazards that may cause an accident. During this visit you'll also receive safety items such as a bathmat, smoke detector, nightlights and more.
· Bids on any safety related project.

Our independent contractors and handymen are screened and fully insured. They will show up on time and do an excellent job at a reasonable price.*

---

* Flyer for Home Safe Home, 2005.

Seitz said, "Older people are more concerned with fires and break-ins....You see a lot of those on TV. When my aunt falls and loses her independence, it'll never make the news. But the sad fact is that more people age 65 and over die from falls than from fires and car accidents combined."[32]

Working first as a volunteer, Seitz soon became an employee and led the program to develop relationships with other organizations and to serve a growing number of the area's seniors. He provided safety education talks to groups all over the region, qualified clients under the same income guidelines, hired contractors and supplied the materials for the larger projects they executed, such as ramps, grab bars and railings.

To further the credibility of the services provided through HSH, Seitz later earned certified aging in place specialist credentials. He also participated in the Executive Certification for Home Modifiers program out of the University of Southern California.

SEEKING PARTNERS AND SUPPORT

Adult Resources requested $30,000 from VCA for HSH in 2002, which led to approval of a $15,000 grant with the condition that an ad hoc committee be formed to explore more permanent funding solutions for this important service. VCA expressed concern over supporting HSH through Adult Resources. The board encouraged HSH to search for a new parent organization. While Adult Resources wanted to keep the program, VCA decided that if no definite plans were made for HSH's future, it would not continue to fund the program.

HSH goals were exceeded at all levels in the second year of VCA's support. However, a proposed budget of $80,000 for 2003, including $15,000 from VCA, would not be enough to cover costs, even though its service potential and impact remained strong. A new committee was formed to help with fundraising, and for a time, partnerships helped to provide financial support.

HSH continued to grow and reach more seniors who needed to make their homes safer. In 2003, 120 projects were completed, an increase over 112 in 2002. In the first eight and a half months of 2004, 1,500 "Home Safety Self-Evaluation Booklets" had been distributed, 125 home safety inspections had been conducted and the program was on track to complete 160 to 175 installations for the year.

Officially Adopted by VCA

When Adult Resources announced it would close on October 31, 2004, VCA considered options for the future of HSH and VCA's support of the organization, including:

- VCA adopting the HSH program versus continuing to provide funding
- The willingness of the Beaver County Office on Aging (BCOA) to continue to provide funding for HSH should VCA become involved
- VCA acting only as a fiduciary pass through for the program
- The possibility of hiring the HSH coordinator as an independent contractor
- The goal of moving HSH services into Allegheny County
- The possibility that VCA might need to fund the program to a greater extent than originally anticipated as the BCOA didn't cover salary, benefits or office expenses
- The legal ramifications and liabilities involved if VCA decided to adopt HSH

At a special meeting on September 29, 2004, the VCA board of trustees approved a resolution to adopt the HSH program from Adult Resources. Adult Resources cancelled its contract with the BCOA, which was rewritten and awarded to VCA. VCA approved an initial grant of $30,000 to fund program operations. Seitz became a full-time employee of VCA on October 1, 2004.

As VCA absorbed HSH, it set goals for 2004–05 to expand into Allegheny County, market and brand HSH as part of VCA, set a fee structure for clients who could pay, recruit more volunteers (possibly from the Masonic Village woodworking shop) and develop standards for projects.

Paying clients were identified as those with monthly income above $1,500. Financial assistance was provided by VCA for those who couldn't afford to pay. Clients in Beaver County who were under the threshold were reimbursed by BCOA under a contract with VCA.

Over the years, HSH established working relationships with other organizations. The SECORO Foundation of Sewickley Savings Bank had been a loyal partner to HSH, providing financial support each year. VCA was

HSH Clients Share Their Gratitude

"Hi, I just wanted to thank you all for the changes you made in my bathroom. I don't know if you understand the problem I had getting up and down. It's only been a week, but it has made a big difference to my life. I thank God for your program. I know it has made a big difference in a lot of people's lives. Keep up the good work."—Lillie C.

"Thank you so much for your personal assistance in helping to make John's house an accessible home again." —Al C.

"I want to thank you so much for getting me my beautiful ramp. You were so kind and courteous to come back and raise the end for me when it was sloped too much for me to handle. It looks good and I am enjoying my new sense of freedom and getting out so much." —Anonymous

"Recently your contractor installed some grab bars in my tub and brought a sturdy bench for the tub. He was exceedingly polite, professional, and compassionate. He deserves a star." —Dora C.

"Thank you and Valley Care Association so much for the ramp. I am so thankful that I can now come out whenever I want. My neighbors are pleased and they all admire it. Most of all my family loves it because it's taken a load off of them." —Nellis S.

Thank you notes printed in the Valley Care newsletter, Fall 2006.

also a subcontractor for Lutheran Service Society, fulfilling the home safety component of a grant received for its Meals on Wheels program.

Another HSH supporter was the Beaver County Office on Aging Community Support Fund, which was available to older adults in Beaver County who weren't required to participate in the full BCOA. The program bypassed red tape to expedite home safety projects. Many such clients were referred by home health agencies who worked with the seniors in their homes. Several years later, in 2008, HSH received a five-year contract from the Community Support Fund.

Volunteer Profile: Conrad and Tom Rehm

Conrad and Tom Rehm started Conrose Maintenance and Repair, a commercial cleaning and maintenance service, in 2000, when they retired from their respective careers. To the benefit of HSH, Conrad and Tom rediscovered their love for working with their hands. From the installation of stair rails, bathroom grab bars and wheelchair ramps, to electrical and plumbing repairs, the Rehms have completed more than forty HSH projects.

"I enjoy meeting the people we help through the Home Safe Home program," said Conrad, a former plant manager of West Penn Plastics in New Castle. "I like to see the relief they experience knowing that we are there to make their home a place where they can continue to live safely. Everyone is so friendly and appreciative."

Tom, a mechanical engineer, built Invia Industries, which specialized in architectural lighting design. "I like nothing better than using my skills to take a difficult situation and make it work for the homeowner," he said.

Expanding Services through Referrals

Over the years that HSH made homes safer and living at home possible for thousands of area seniors, the program gained wide name recognition in Allegheny and Beaver Counties. Referrals came from government and community agencies, various health care providers, health insurance plans and former clients and their families.

In 2006, HSH also met with Lowe's home improvement stores, whose volunteers had supported the program under Adult Resources. Lowe's made plans to distribute a new self-guided workbook. That same year, HSH held discussions with LIFE Beaver to explore opportunities to provide services.

Becoming Part of the VCA Strategic Plan

Over the years, HSH became more sophisticated in marketing and delivering services. A strategic plan was developed in 2007 to dovetail with VCA's strategies for the next eighteen to twenty-four months. Its primary goal was to "provide excellent home safety services while exploring new revenue streams and collaborative opportunities in order to expand program capacity while keeping costs to a minimum."

HSH developed activities to pursue each of its three strategies:

1. Strengthen impact through collaborations, partnerships and education, by:
   - Seeking partners and opportunities for collaboration
   - Strengthening relationships with Sewickley Savings Bank/ SECORO Foundation
   - Broadening community and professional understanding of HSH
2. Streamline program procedures to:
   - Simplify purchasing process
   - Move the inventory and the program coordinator to same location
   - Maximize use of volunteers
   - Create a VCA volunteer program
3. Increase HSH visibility to expand public knowledge of home safety and HSH services through extensive community outreach.

Throughout 2007, HSH worked on a reorganization plan for its operations, searched for a volunteer to assist the coordinator and looked for ways to make the program more sustainable. In 2008, it introduced a falls assessment screening tool.

Beginning in 2009, HSH began an association with the Rebuilding Together program, a national non-profit that enlisted professionals to volunteer to make building improvements for low-income seniors. The group's largest event was Rebuilding Day on the last Saturday of April. Working with the local affiliate, Rebuilding Together Pittsburgh, the SECORO Foundation sponsored several homes to be refurbished each year as part of this event.

STATE GRANT ENABLES PROGRAM EXPANSION

In 2011, HSH was one of five organizations statewide to receive a Home Modification Construction Officer (HMCO) pilot program expansion grant, which helped adults who received in-home support through state and federal funds to remain living at home for as long as possible. The grant was awarded by the Pennsylvania Department of Public Welfare's office of long-term living and was administered by the Pennsylvania Housing Finance Agency.

HOME SAFE HOME SWOT (DECEMBER 2007)

STRENGTHS

- Educated and committed board and committee
- The aging services network regionally and statewide is becoming familiar with VCA and programs
- HSH meets an unmet need
- Falls prevention and home safety are huge on national radar screen
- Program's successful track record
- VCA/HSH positive reputation
- VCA has financial resources sufficient to support HSH
- VCA is good at partnering with other organizations
- Affluent service area
- Strong relationship with SECORO Foundation

WEAKNESSES

- Program is not financially independent
- Program procedural processes need work, i.e., reducing number of vendors, finding adequate storage for inventory
- Program is currently at capacity for one staff (225–230 projects per year)
- Inconsistent marketing due to insufficient staff
- Insufficient fundraising strategies
- Vulnerability of VCA funds to investment market fluctuations
- Insufficient community support
- No "professional" information and referral (I & R) for clients, many of whom could benefit from additional services
- Limited service area
- Limited project funding

OPPORTUNITIES

- Current trend to increase services for elderly in the community rather than in the nursing home
- Aging demographics brings rise in demand for home and community-based services

- Consistent expression by elders that their desire is to age in place
- VCA/HSH strong networking and connections with aging services provider network
- Sewickley is a community that is committed to serving its residents
- Large number of local companies with many employees caring for an elderly loved one that could use services
- Home health agencies as partners
- Public knowledge of the program is still limited and has potential for growth

THREATS
- Shrinking public monies
- Government funders in flux, and funding most likely to decrease (BCOA community fund may disappear)
- Local economy is unstable Competition for donations (particularly in Sewickley) is high
- VCA investments static
- HSH prices generally higher than private contractor fees (we need to add on our percent)
- High cost of general and professional liability

The state created the HMCO program to promote the underused waiver funds for home modifications and to increase the number of home modification professionals throughout the state. Waiver funds were provided by the state to those who qualified for huge projects, such as bathrooms, and required more paperwork and approval.

The first HMCO grant award was $87,500 for the first six months of 2011, with the possibility of a full-year renewal for $150,000. Participation in the pilot required HSH to expand into Lawrence County and to service all adults who received state-funded services to enable them to remain at home. At the successful completion of the pilot, HSH's grants were renewed for the next two years, enabling it to secure a full-time home modification construction officer for the remainder of the grant period.

CLIENT PROFILES: TOM AND KATE HORNSTEIN

The goal of seniors like Tom and Kate Hornstein of Moon Township was to remain living in their home safely and independently for as long as they were able. As they aged, they knew they would need to make home modifications.

After Tom broke his hip, Kate called Valley Care Association's Home Safe Home program and arranged to have a home safety inspection. "We did a couple of obvious things such as getting a lift chair and a stair glide, but the great value of Home Safe Home for us was having a professional look at the safety of our home," Kate said. "We felt that we could use an impartial eye to do a walk-through inspection because they would see things that we would not. John [Seitz] was easily able to spot a half dozen potentially dangerous areas that never even occurred to us, for instance, because Tom has a walker he asked, 'Did you notice that your sidewalk cuts out strangely right at the end of the port?' He came up with recommendations for things that had never crossed our minds."*

---

* *Valley Care Newsletter*, Spring 2008.

NEW OPPORTUNITIES FOR GROWTH

While there were opportunities to expand the HSH service area in 2012 through Allegheny and Butler Counties, funding began to shift. The BCOA reduced the HSH budget by 50 percent, causing HSH to search for small, fee-for-service projects and create a waiting list for subsidized work.

Seitz helped design the accessible garden at the Ambridge ADS site and was approached by Home Depot to help create additional accessible gardens at other care facilities, including Sunnyview in Butler, Saint Barnabas, Passavant, Vincentian Homes, Kane-Scott, Kane-Ross, the Willows and Washington County Health Center. The gardens were completed with the help of Home Depot, which also printed one thousand color copies of the "Self-Guided Home Safety" workbook to be distributed at marketing events and presentations.

With the HMCO grant ending in June 2013, HSH looked for an additional $50,000 in grants to supplement the $60,000 from the BCOA. Because it was so difficult for this type of program to be self-sustaining, VCA considered keeping HSH as one of its own programs.

A NEW ERA UNDER LUTHERAN SENIORLIFE

When VCA signed an agreement with Lutheran SeniorLife in 2013, both Adult Day Services and HSH moved to LSL. LSL considered whether the HSH program was sustainable beyond the three-year funding in the affiliation agreement. In August, Matt Long, the HMCO, accepted a position at LSL on a contract basis. Seitz followed him to LSL later that year.

Ultimately, HSH was moved under Visiting Nurses Association, Western Pennsylvania, another member of the LSL family. VCA continued to provide funding, with the Visiting Nurses Association receiving a management fee to run the program at an executive level.

BOARD MEMBER PROFILE: JAMES R. LAMPERSKI

James R. Lamperski, CFP, joined the Valley Care Endowment Board in 2010. This was just three years after VCE was established as a separate corporation in charge of managing the investment portfolio and distributing funds for the benefit of the Valley Care Association. He became president of the VCE board in 2016, serving until 2019.

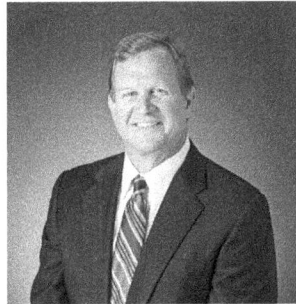

James R. Lamperski, CFP.
Courtesy of Valley Care Association.

Lamperski directed the organization through its transition from directly managing elder care services to primarily providing financial support to Lutheran SeniorLife as it managed Home Safe Home and Adult Day Services. He also led efforts to preserve the endowment, seek new opportunities for VCA and chronicle the organization's history.

Lamperski is a professional financial planner and investment advisor. Since July 2008, he has been senior director, senior wealth manager and vice president at the Bank of New York Mellon, Pittsburgh. He previously served as a financial consultant at Teachers Insurance and Annuity Association—College Retirement Equities Fund (TIAA CREF) and at Smith Barney of Citigroup.

A 1990 graduate of the Indiana University of Pennsylvania, he gained certification in financial planning in 1995. Lamperski lives in Ohio Township with his wife, Rebecca, and two daughters, Jessica and Jackie.

MAKING SENIORS' APARTMENTS SAFER

After undergoing two knee replacements, Jean Harvey, eighty-four, was happy to know that modifications being made in her apartment's bathroom would help make life easier and safer. Harvey, who had lived in the Union Aid Society apartments in Sewickley for fifteen years, wasn't the only resident excited for the new updates.

Helen Rondinelli, eighty-one, the longest resident after nineteen years, agreed the safety modifications were much appreciated. "We needed it," Rondinelli said, "and it will be wonderful."

Three Sewickley-based non-profits—Valley Care Association, the Union Aid Society and the SECORO Foundation—joined forces in 2012 for a one-day home improvement blitz at the twenty-two apartments within the Union Aid buildings at 511 Centennial Avenue. Union Aid provides affordable apartments for low-income older adults who have ties to Quaker Valley School District communities.

The project's objective was to help keep those older residents safe in their homes by making shower and toilet modifications. The home installations included forty-four shower grab bars and six elevated toilets that are easier for residents to get on and off.

"It's been a wonderful example of neighbors helping neighbors," Seitz said, pointing out that the four contractors—three from Beaver County and one from Carnegie—were also working together.

Secoro had worked with Valley Care for many years, but it was the first time they'd ever done a renovation through Union Aid Society.[*]

---

[*] Larissa Dudkiewicz, "Patch Staff," Sewickley Patch, November 9, 2012, https://patch.com.

Susan Nirschel, director of Valley Care Adult Day Services, who helps to oversee HSH, explained that "HSH covers Allegheny, Armstrong, Beaver, Butler, and Lawrence counties. VCA is now in an advisory role, but it's the LSL board that ultimately makes final decisions concerning HSH. The move helped Valley Care to remain sustainable."

The change was considered strategic in that the two organizations are like-minded, and HSH benefited from the marketing efforts and visibility of the Visiting Nurses Association. As a result, HSH reported growth in 2014, including a 57 percent increase in home safety inspections and a 10 percent increase in completed projects, such as ramps, easy-step tubs and stair lifts.

With the BCOA increasing funding to $120,000 at the end of 2014, HSH added a full-time and a part-time employee to assist Seitz. Activity remained brisk in Beaver County with some activity in Allegheny and Butler Counties. Secoro funding picked up within its service area, and a number of private pay projects continued.

Seitz retired on October 31, 2016, after fourteen years with HSH. "John was so committed and worked hard," said Deb Shtulman, executive director of VCA. "He put his stamp on the program and really wanted to support seniors in their environment—enabling them to stay at home."

Carlo DelTurco, previously an HSH contractor, was named program coordinator in January 2017. "With funding moving to the managed care model, we are in the middle of the process of figuring out how to work with the insurance companies and who to use," he said. "We still get some private pay, but we're looking hard for new funding."

There's no place like home. Keep yours safe and accessible.
—*Lutheran SeniorLife*

Epilogue

DECIDING ON THE FUTURE
OF VALLEY CARE

Throughout its history, Valley Care Association (VCA), including the Valley Care Endowment (VCE), has remained true to its mission and the people in the community it has served. This commitment guided the strategic adjustments made over the years to remain a viable and sustainable organization in the face of evolving needs and changes in health care and human services trends and reimbursements.

In the first forty years, these adjustments led to three distinct phases of operation, each focused on the demographic, economic and human services realities of the time:

1. The initial formation of VCA and the development and operation of the Valley Care Nursing Home and Adult Day Care Centers
2. The sale of the nursing home to Masonic Village, shifting VCA's activity to grant-making, Home Safe Home and adult day services
3. Partnering with Lutheran SeniorLife to manage and take responsibility for the two VCA Adult Day Services facilities and Home Safe Home.

Early in 2018, the boards of all three organizations (VCA, VCE and LSL) realized that they were facing yet more changes. Pressure within the health care industry reduced reimbursements for ADS, leaving families without the financial support needed to pay for services that keep seniors healthy, mentally engaged, socially involved and out of nursing homes. Further, the delivery of care was shifting from institution-based services and medical models toward aging at home (or aging in place) and dementia services. As a result, adult day care facilities experienced reduced attendance, and many were closing.

Would these events serve as the catalyst for another iteration?

CONSIDERING A VARIETY OF OPTIONS

In anticipation of the next phase of the story, the VCA, VCE and LSL boards began working together to identify the emerging and unmet needs of the aging population, strategize how to meet those needs and recommend solutions. A committee was formed to explore and research options for VCA to provide new services for senior citizens in the service area. Among the possible solutions were:

- Continue total or partial financial support of LSL as it serves the elderly through ADS
- Return to a grant-making strategy to support community-based initiatives
- Support emerging digital options and other technologies that enhance the aging-at-home experience
- Develop a referral service to coordinate care and provide information about existing services for seniors
- Support a mix of these concepts

The committee evaluated the ADS model, including enrollment, participant acuity, referral and payor sources and disenrollment. To fully study the idea of a referral service to connect seniors to care and support, it also conducted a community-needs assessment; developed a program description and scope of services; identified the geographic service area; and drafted job descriptions, implementation steps and outcome measures.

CONSOLIDATING ADS

Even as the boards processed the committee's findings to determine next steps, LSL and VCA agreed to close the Moon ADS in Cherrington in April 2019, following years of attendance at less than capacity, the retirement of Executive Director Susan Nirschel and the departure of other key staff members. Most employees took positions elsewhere within LSL. Several of the Moon ADS clients began attending the Ambridge program.

"At this point, privately funded and operated day care does not seem to be viable [in the long run]," said VCE board member Bill Ringle. "It appears to be more viable if it is linked physically and financially to a medical facility or a center with other services for seniors, rather than a 'stand-alone' as our centers are."

VCE continued to support the LSL/ADS initiative in Ambridge while determining a viable role for this service.

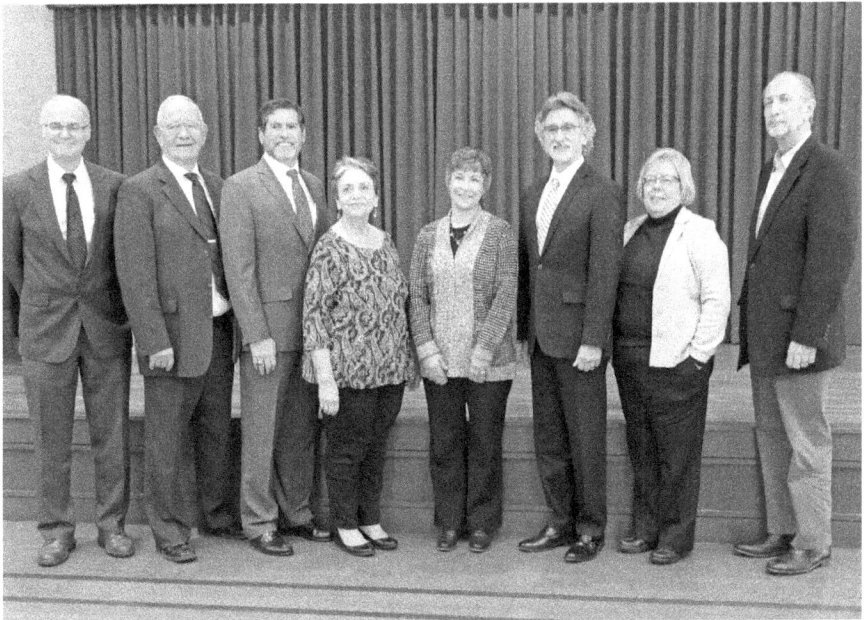

VCA board members Dr. Chris O'Donnell, Brandon James, David Fair, Janice Wendt, Donna Van Kirk, Joseph M. Olimpi, Elizabeth Moore and Terry Mann. *Courtesy of Valley Care Association.*

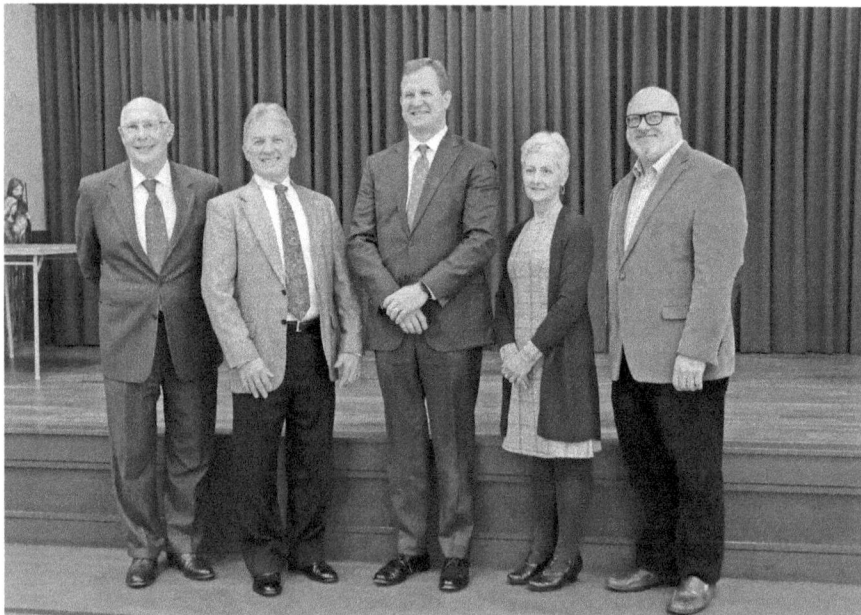

VCE board members Dr. Dan Brooks, Bill Ringle, Jamie Lamperski, Regan Fetterolf and Dr. Dick Hogan. *Courtesy of Valley Care Association.*

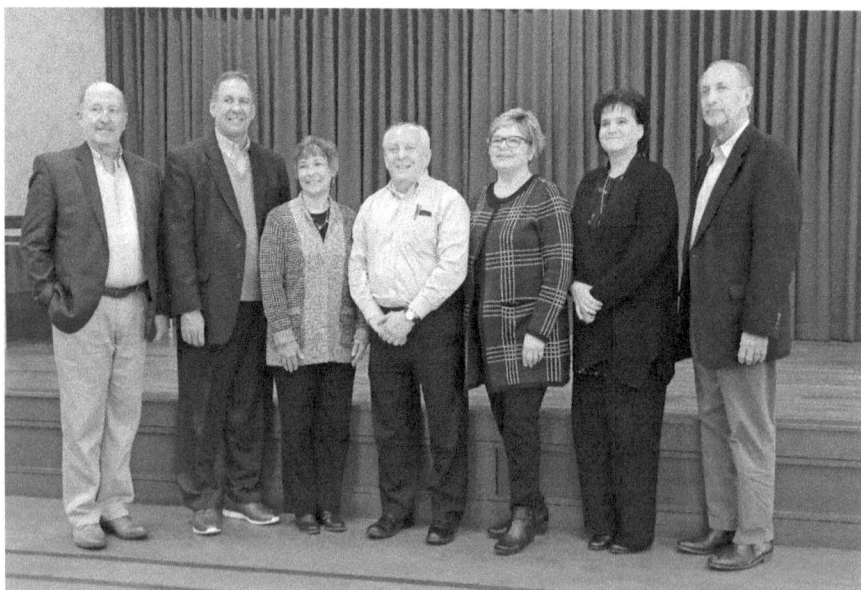

Lutheran SeniorLife board members Jeff Carraway, David J. Fenoglietto, Donna Van Kirk, David Hamm, Susan Nirschel, Caroline Robaskiwicz and Terry Mann. *Courtesy of Valley Care Association.*

A Disciplined Process to Determine the Future

Whatever decisions are made concerning future services, the organizations involved are committed to following the same prudent evaluation process that proved successful when reaching crossroads in the past. "To determine what direction VCA should take in the current environment, we are going back to the beginning, following the methods used in founding our organization," said VCE board president Jamie Lamperski. "We have the benefit of their road map and intend to follow it."

That roadmap includes three key components:

1. Focusing on the fundamental mission and operational principles
2. Answering the question, "Is this in line with what the founders intended?"
3. Engaging well-respected consultants and experts to gather data, offer conclusions and make recommendations

Among the questions the consultants and experts will be asked to consider are:

- Who are the potential clients and what are their needs?
- Should the social determinants of health drive future strategies and tactics?
- Should community organizations be engaged in the discussion as they were at the beginning in 1978?
- Is the VCE foundation large enough to make a difference in today's world, or should a philanthropic partner be identified, and what scale is necessary to remain relevant while preserving capital?
- What is the potential to raise significant funds, if necessary?

The Valley Care boards' diligent and careful stewardship of resources over the last forty years made it possible to navigate change and continue to serve seniors. It's this diligent and methodical oversight that will guide the boards in making the decisions necessary to deliver innovative and successful human services programs for seniors in the years to come.

As this book goes to press, the future direction of VCA remains open to many possibilities. The only certainty is that it will continue to use its resources, the focus of its mission and the dedication of its board members to benefit the elderly in the Sewickley Valley.

Epilogue

When Valley Care ran things, if you needed something you got it. If it was valuable for the clients, they would find a way to get it. We had a very devoted group of people who really wanted that to work. As I look back, the highlight was that I learned how to get along with the aged. I learned how to be humble by watching people take care of [the elderly] *and people with dementia. I also learned why you need to give back—it's that when you help other people you recognize that one day this could be you. And you hope that someday someone is going to be there to help you.*

—*Gwen Ogle*

APPENDIX

MEMBERS OF THE BOARD OF DIRECTORS OF VALLEY CARE ASSOCIATION*

LAST NAME	FIRST NAME	FIRST YEAR OF TERM	LAST YEAR OF TERM	LEADERSHIP POSITIONS
Addison	James	1993	1995	
Alexander	James H.	1984	2004	President 1992–93 and 1999
Armstrong	John A.	1986	1990	
Beall	Frank	1978	1980	
Bell	Arlene	2015	2024	
Benz	Ralph	1978	1987	
Bikowski, MD	Joseph B.	1981	1988	
Bobonis, Sr.	Regis D	2002	2002	
Boswell	William	1990	1997	
Brooks, MD	Daniel H.	2008	2013	President, 2012
Carton	Mrs. P.D.	1994	1996	
Cheponis, MD	George	1985	1988	
Clarke, MD	Charles E.	1983	1985	
Colbert	Elizabeth "Betty"	1978	1990	

Last Name	First Name	First Year of Term	Last Year of Term	Leadership Positions
Cooper	C. William	1986	1990	
Cooper	James	1994	1999	
Coward, MD	Holly Jean	1998	1998	
Curry	William C	2008	2013	
Denardo	Sharon	2015	2024	
Deutsch	Clayton	1987	1989	
Devens	Henry F.	1985	1986	
Dewhirst	Jeffrey	1985	1990	
Doebler, MD	Robert	1993	1997	
Duggan	R.D. "Bob"	1978	1980	
Edson	John Jay	2000	2010	
Evansky	Reverend William J.	2000	2006	
Fadzen	Karen F.	2002	2007	
Fair	David A.	2015	2024	
Farina	Reverend Edward R.	1981	1985	
Ferguson	J. Robert	1980	1996	President, 1981–87
Flannery	Charles	2005		
Flannery	Kevin M.	2008	2013	
Fletcher	Charles	1999	2007	
Ford	Carole Moore	2008	2013	
Forsyth	Margaret	1991	1995	
Fortunato	Michael V.	2005	2013	
Foster	John K.	1983	1985	
Franks	B.J.	1998	2008	
Gartner	Elinor O.	1983	1985	

Last Name	First Name	First Year of Term	Last Year of Term	Leadership Positions
Gartner	Rodney W.	2002	2007	
Gordon	Herb	1998	2003	
Gross	Eric	2011	2020	President, 2017–2020
Harper	Matrid	1998	2006	
Haver, MD	Paul M.	1982	1983	
Hay	Thomas S.	2000	2001	
Hays	Alice	1978	1987	
Heinlen	Calvin X.	1978	1987	
Hess	Peggy	1988	1991	
Hess	Thomas D.	1988	1991	
Hess, Jr.	Raymond L.	1981	1985	
Hickox	Paul	1978	1983	
Hogan	Linda	2017	2026	
Hyatt	Cheryl A.	2006	2013	
James, MD	Edward E.	1978	1982	
James	R. Brandon	2014	2023	
Jehle	Michael	1998	2000	
Jones, III	Betty	1978	1981	
Kelley	Linda J.	2004	2012	
Kelly	William	1989	1991	
King	Jane	1978	1984	
Ludwig, MD	Karl D.	1981	1992	
March	Betty	1984	1985	
March	Eugene	1982	1992	
March	Gene	1998	2000	
Marsh	Gertrude	1989	1991	
Marshall, DO	Lonnie	1993	1995	
McClester	Jean	1995	1999	

Last Name	First Name	First Year of Term	Last Year of Term	Leadership Positions
McClester	John R.	1989	1991	
McKibbin	Kay	1988	1988	
Meenan	Rev. Joseph S.	1986	1988	
Merrill, Jr.	Nancy	1986	1990	
Michael	Linda Rice	1998	2006	
Montgomery, Jr.	Edward A.	1984	1985	
Moore	Elizabeth "Libby"	2009	2018	
Morgan	Paula	1989	1990	
Mullaugh	Carol	1993	1997	
Nadler	Patty	1989	1990	
Nash	Rody	2008	2012	
Nash	Stephen	1994	1995	
Neely, Jr.	T.W.	1978	1987	
Nelson	Wayne	1995	1997	
Nimick	David A.	1978	1985	
O'Donnell, MD	Chris	2017	2026	
Ogle	Gwendolyn M.	1991	2008	
Olimpi, Esq.	Joseph M.	2018	2027	
Pearson	Nathan W.	1978	1987	
Peters	Daniel E.	2003	2012	President, 2008
Phipps	Anne G.	1993	2000	
Purvis	Robert	2007	2013	
Ramsburg	Virginia "Deedo"	1978	1989	
Ramsey	Paul D.	1978	1985	
Ranson	J.P. "John"	1993	1997	

Last Name	First Name	First Year of Term	Last Year of Term	Leadership Positions
Rideout	Vike	1998	2000	
Ringle	Lorena M.	2015	2024	
Ringle	William L.	2007	2013	
Roller, RN	Lori	2017	2026	
Ronaldson, MD	Agnes	1978		
Ross	Carl A.	2012	2013	
Ryan	Dale	1983	1987	
Schroeder	Charlotte B.	1978	1990	
Schulenburg (Miller)	Wenda Lee	2000	2008	President, 2004–2007
Selkovits, MD	Sidney	1978	1984	
Semple	Phyllis K.	1986	1989	
Shoop, Sr.	Richard	1982	1983	
Smith	Barbara	1983	1989	
Smith	Warren L.	1982	1985	
Snyder	G. Whitney	1978	1989	
Snyder	Jean S.	1989	1990	
Speak	H. Alan	1978	1981	
States	James H.	1978	1980	
Still	Reverend Walter C.	1985		
Stone	Laura	1992	1997	
Theys	Jim	1999	2004	President, 2002–2003
Thomas	Cynthia Church	2008	2017	President, 2016–2017
Thompson	LeRoy	1986	1989	
Toliver	Reverend Jezreel	1978	1985	
Trainer	Mrs. John M.	1982	1985	

Last Name	First Name	First Year of Term	Last Year of Term	Leadership Positions
Tumpson	Jane	1995	1999	President, 1997–98
Turner, III	Reverend Russell W.	1978	1981	
Urda	Karl J.	1983	1990	
Vales	Joseph	1992	1997	
Walsh, PhD	Ruth Laird	2002	2004	
Walter	Elizabeth	1978	1983	
Wedeen	Marvin	1978	2008	President, 1993–96
Wendt, III	J. Scott	1984	1990	
Wilcock	Catherine C.	1993	1995	
Yost	Mrs. James	1982	1983	
Zacharias	Helen	1992	2003	

*This list of board members and their terms was compiled according to available records. Some records were incomplete and others may have been missing.

MEMBERS OF THE BOARD OF DIRECTORS OF VALLEY CARE ENDOWMENT

Last Name	First Name	First Year of Term	Last Year of Term	Leadership Positions
Bell	Arlene	2016		
Brooks, MD	Daniel E.	2014		
Cawley	Kraig	2010	2014	
DiNuzzo	P.J.	2011	2012	
Fadzen	Karen F.	2007	2010	
Hogan, MD	Richard	2015		
Lamperski	James	2010	2019	President, 2016
Michael	Linda Rice	2007	2012	
Peters	Daniel E.	2007	2012	President, 2007

Last Name	First Name	First Year of Term	Last Year of Term	Leadership Positions
Purvis	Robert	2007	2012	
Ringle	William	2014		
Thomas	Cynthia Church	2016	2017	

Directors of VCA Adult Day Care Center or Adult Day Services

Last Name	First Name	Starting Year	Final Year
Pritchard	Janice L.	1983	1984
Benefield	Carole A.	1984	1985
Miller	Kathi	1985	1989
Fortunato*	Michael	1989	1989
Ciocarello	James	1989	1997
Rosequist, RN	Mark	1997	1998
Lelinksi	Mary	1998	1999
Carr	Jennifer	1999	2004
Shtulman**	Deb	2001	2008
Hostutler***	Debbie	2007	2009
Sedlacko	Heather	2008	2013
Nirschel	Susan	2012	2019

*interim director
** executive director of VCA, with a primary role as director of adult day services
*** program coordinator in Ambridge, then Cherrington

VCA Directors and Executive Directors

Last Name	First Name	Years
Moore	Betts (Elizabeth G.)	1981–86
Hamren	Marcia	1986–88
Martinez	Diane	1988–92
Tumpson	Jane	1999–2001
Shtulman	Deborah	2001–2008
Sedlacko	Heather	2008–2013

VALLEY CARE AUXILIARY PRESIDENTS

LAST NAME	FIRST NAME	YEARS
Ryan	Dale	1985–86
McKibbin	Kay	1987
Hess	Peggy	1988–89
Snow	Diane	1990
Ogle	Gwen	1991, 1993
Carton	Pat	1992, 1994–95
Lessman	Ruth	1996–99

GRANTS AWARDED BY VALLEY CARE ASSOCIATION

- Adult Resources to support Home Safe Home for two years with a potential match for a third year
- Adult Resources and Sweetwater Center for the Arts for an intergenerational art project with fourth graders and older adults; intergenerational art project in middle schools
- Adult Resources for the purchase of a new building
- Alzheimer's Association for the Safe Return Program, which issued ID bracelets to ensure the safe return of people who wander from home or become lost
- Beaver County Office on Aging to launch the *Beaver County Senior News*
- Beaver County Office on Aging to create the Rest and Relaxation (R&R) program for caregiver respite in cooperation with Homemakers and Home Health Aides of Beaver County
- *Beaver County Senior News* to underwrite a half-page monthly column focused on volunteer recruitment
- Better Than Ever Independents, a senior acting company
- Center for Hope for Bridging the Gap multi-generational program to pair adults fifty and older with at-risk children in the Ambridge area
- Center of Hope's Lunch and Learn programs for older adults in Ambridge and the surrounding communities
- Comprehensive Service Alliance for caregiver training workshops and support to enable older adults with mental retardation to age in place

- Contact Pittsburgh for a daily telephone reassurance service for older adults recently discharged from the hospital or who lived alone and were isolated and/or frail
- Crisis Center North for Domestic Violence in Later Life Project
- ElderCare Coalition to print thirteen thousand copies of the "Help Yourself Resource Guide" that listed resources for older adults
- Faith in Action program of the Sewickley Valley YMCA to alleviate the loneliness and frustration of advancing age
- Generations Together for GrandKIN Raising GrandKIDS program to conduct needs assessment for a parenting grandparent support group, intergenerational activities; a garden project for students and VCA ADS clients
- Heritage Valley Health System's Independence for Over Eighty Initiative, the only hospital-supported initiative in Western Pennsylvania, which provided case management home visits, as well as education on advance directives, reduced hospital readmissions and encouraged medication compliance
- Heritage Valley Health System and Sewickley Valley Hospital for Community Advanced Illness Program to provide outreach, information and education to African American communities for advanced care planning
- LifeSpan Incorporated for study on recommendations for future senior services
- Lutheran Affiliated Services to fund caregiver tract at its seventh-annual Conference on Successful Aging and for a scholarship fund
- Lutheran Service Society's Meals on Wheels program to update and repair equipment in the Sewickley Valley area kitchens that prepared meals that were delivered to the frail and elderly
- Passavant Memorial Homes, the parent of Comprehensive Services Alliance, for training workshops for professional and personal caregivers to be held at the VCA Adult Day Services site
- Presbyterian SeniorCare for publication of educational materials ("A Guide to Living and Care Options") for town meetings
- Project for Love, a group of seniors who make free turbans and pillows for cancer patients
- Retired Senior Volunteer Program

- Sewickley Valley YMCA's Faith in Action (later renamed Ohio Valley Neighbors in Action) to underwrite the annual holiday concert with the River City Brass Band with proceeds to benefit Faith in Action
- SWPA Partnership for Aging for the Let Your Voice Be Heard project to provide focus groups and information gathering
- VCA Adult Day Services for creative arts therapy program
- Valley Care Masonic Center for production and distribution of senior services referral directory
- Valley Care Adult Day Services to support the cost of operations
- Valley Care Masonic Center for the Financial Assistance for Assisted Living Fund for those who met the criteria
- The Arc of Beaver County for the third-annual A Better End seminar
- Union Aid Society to renovate two apartment buildings and add elevators
- Villa Saint Joseph's Building on God's Great Love Campaign
- Western Regional Wisdom Center, a collaborative program of the Lutheran Service Society, the Sewickley YMCA and Adult Resources for a "center without walls" with activities in multiple locations—launched at the Mall at Robinson in Allegheny County

NOTES

Chapter 1

1. "Sewickley in a Hurry," Sewickley Valley Historical Society, 2001, https://www.sewickleyhistory.org.
2. "Sewickley History," Sewickley Valley Historical Society, https://www.sewickleyhistory.org.
3. Union Aid Society.
4. *Sewickley Herald*, June 14, 1951.
5. Ibid., September 27, 1951.
6. Centers for Medicare and Medicaid Services, *National Health Expenditures 2017 Highlights*, 2017, https://www.cms.gov.
7. Katharine R. Levit et al., "National Health Expenditures, 1990," National Center for Biotechnology Information, U.S. National Library of Medicine, https://www.ncbi.nlm.nih.gov.
8. Kate A. Stewart, David C. Grabowski and Darius N. Lakdawalla, "Annual Expenditures for Nursing Home Care: Private and Public Payer Price Growth, 1977–2004," *Med Care* 47, no. 3 (March 2009): 295–301, https://insights.ovid.com.
9. Kaiser Family Foundation, "Medicaid's Role in Nursing Home Care," June 20, 2017, https://www.kff.org.

Chapter 2

10. Ibid., February 18, 1981.
11. Mike May, "Sewickley Woman's Dream 50 Years Later," *Sewickley Herald*, June 24, 1987.
12. *Sewickley Herald*, September 28, 1983.
13. Ibid., March 7, 1984.

Chapter 3

14. Ibid., November 11, 1981.
15. Ibid., March 14, 1984.
16. *Beaver County Times*, December 16, 1985.
17. *Pittsburgh Post-Gazette North*, April 5, 1984.

Chapter 4

18. *Beaver/Allegheny Times*, October 24, 1981.

Chapter 6

19. *Sewickley Herald*, January 23, 1985.
20. Ibid., April 3, 1985.
21. Ibid.
22. *Valley Care Update Newsletter*, Summer 1989.
23. *Pennsylvania Freemason Magazine*, May 1999.
24. "Retirement Living Minutes from Pittsburgh," Masonic Villages, https://masonicvillages.org.

Chapter 7

25. Valley Care Association Board Minutes.
26. *Beaver County Times*, July 13, 1983.
27. Ibid.
28. *Valley Care Newsletter*, 1988.

29. *Beaver County Times,* June 24, 1993.
30. *Valley Cares Newsletter*, 2011.
31. Ibid.

Chapter 9

32. *Sewickley Herald*, 2001.

BIBLIOGRAPHY

Archives

Sewickley Herald Digital Archive. Sewickley Public Library, Sewickley, PA.
   http://sewickleylibrary.org.

News

Beaver County/Allegheny Times
Care Connection Valley Care Association Newsletter, 1987–2000
Pittsburgh Post-Gazette
Valley Cares Newsletter, 2005–10
Valley Care Update Newsletter, 1985–86

Reports

Annual Reports of Valley Care Association, 1984–2004.
Gaynes, Neil L., principal consultant; Donovan Gardner, senior consultant;
   and Susan J. Morse, director of planning. *Comprehensive Planning Study for
   Valley Care Association*. Sewickley, PA, December 1979.
Katz, Rosalyn. *A Study of Adult Day Care Needs and Demand in Allegheny County, PA.*
   Pittsburgh, PA: Health and Welfare Planning Association of Pittsburgh,
   1981.

Minutes of the Valley Care Executive Committee, Operations Committee and Board of Directors, 1977 to 2018.

Proposal to Staunton Farm from Valley Care, June 1981.

Union Aid Society 100 Years Annual Reports and Minutes, 1898–1998.

Valley Care Appeal for Support with Progress to Date, 1983.

VCA Auxiliary Minutes and Correspondence, 1984–92.

About the Authors

Janice Jeletic has lived her entire life within a few miles of Sewickley. Her marketing and communications career has focused on financial services, consulting, healthcare and higher education. She devotes her free time to volunteer work through her church and community-based organizations that improve the quality of life for local residents in the North Boros of Pittsburgh.

Alison Conte has lived in the Sewickley area for thirty years and enjoys researching and writing about the region's history. A former employee of Sewickley Valley Hospital and the *Sewickley Herald*, she currently works in health care marketing. She published her first novel, *Beyond Normal*, in 2016. Alison spends any free time with her husband, daughter, son-in-law and granddaughter, Violet.

Visit us at
www.historypress.com

www.ingramcontent.com/pod-product-compliance
Lightning Source LLC
Chambersburg PA
CBHW040137270326
41927CB00020B/3423

9 7 8 1 4 6 7 1 4 3 4 2 4